THE DOUBLE ENERGY DIET

JUDI ZUCKER

SHARI ZUCKER

BOOK PUBLISHING COMPANY

Summertown, Tennessee

Library of Congress Cataloging-in-Publication Data

Zucker, Judi.
   The double energy diet : improve your health and vitality— naturally / by
Judi Zucker and Shari Zucker ; endorsed by Earl Mindell and Richard Handin.
     p. cm.
   Includes bibliographical references and index.
   ISBN 978-1-57067-226-2
   1. Health. 2. Nutrition. 3. Exercise. I. Zucker, Shari. II. Title.
RA776.Z83 2008
613—dc22

                 2008008523

© 2008 Judi Zucker and Shari Zucker
Cover and Interior Design: John Wincek
Front and Back Cover Photos: Kenji Photography
Interior Photos: Medeighnia Lentz Photography

Published by
Book Publishing Company
P.O. Box 99
Summertown, TN 38483
1-888-260-8458
www.bookpubco.com

Printed in Canada

ISBN 13 978-1-57067-226-2

14 13 12 11 10 09 08   7 6 5 4 3 2 1

Book Publishing Company is a member
of Green Press Initiative. We chose to print
this title on paper with postconsumer
recycled content and processed chlorine
free, which saved the following natural
resources:

64 trees

3,017 pounds of solid waste

23,494 gallons of water

5,600 pounds pounds of greenhouse gases

45 million BTUs of total energy

For more information, visit
www.greenpressinitiative.org.

*(Paper calculations from Environmental Defense
Paper Calculator: www.papercalculator.org)*

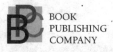 BOOK PUBLISHING COMPANY

 green press INITIATIVE

Contents

EASY ENERGIZING RECIPES

A FEW BASICS

Foreword

by Earl Mindell

I first met Judi and Shari, the "Double-Energy Twins," back in 1979 when they were still in high school and riding high on the success of their first book, *How to Survive Snack Attacks . . . Naturally.*

What impressed me most about the twins was their creativity and vitality—qualities that have matured with them over the years. Judi and Shari have developed their expertise in cooking techniques and their firm grasp of nutritional principles.

The Double Energy Diet describes not just a sound, sensible nutritional program, but a whole way of enriching and enjoying life.

Certainly the twins exemplify this exhilarating Santa Barbara lifestyle. They live it—and they happily share it with you in this invaluable collection of nutritional tips and recipes geared for people of all ages.

Judi and Shari don't believe in complicated cooking techniques or impossible-to-find ingredients. They make their recipes simple to cook and delicious to eat. *The Double Energy Diet* has no gimmicks. It simply encourages a pure, natural way of enjoying fresh, whole foods that will promote good health and high energy.

How lucky we are that Judi and Shari are willing to show us how, with little effort, we can double our energy—and even double our joy in being alive. Here's 2 health!

Earl Mindell, PhD, author of *Dr. Earl Mindell's Natural Remedies for 150 Ailments, Earl Mindell's New Vitamin Bible, Earl Mindell's New Herb Bible, Earl Mindell's Supplement Bible, Earl Mindell's Food as Medicine, Prescription Alternatives, Dr. Earl Mindell's Unsafe at Any Meal, Dr. Earl Mindell's Complete Guide to Natural Cures,* and *Earl Mindell's Peak Performance Bible*

Acknowledgments

Judi: I would like to thank my family for their love, support and encouragement. It's a joy to share a commitment to health and nutrition with my writing partner, Shari. Thanks to Shari for being the best twin sister anyone could ever have—I love you more than words! Thanks to my loving and kind husband, Chris. Thanks to my sweet, smart and passionate children, Taryn and Tanner, for constantly inspiring me. Thank you to my supportive parents, Devra and Irwin Zucker. Mom, you are generous, loving and beautiful. Dad, you are promotion in motion and I appreciate your endless energy! Thanks to our sister, Lori, and Grandmother, Nanz. Thanks to all our family members.

Thanks to Lori Hafner, Jane Henning, Jo Saxon, Dee Nokes, Kathryn Pieron, Lee Scheuermann, Susie and Mark DaRe, Greg Young, Valerie Kendrick, Heidi Waitley and Dawn Darien for their love and friendship.

Shari: I am blessed to have supportive family and friends. I want to acknowledge my family for the lessons they have taught me. Judi has taught me that believing in yourself, working smart, and sheer perseverance will get you what you want in life. Being a twin reinforces the idea of synergy, where the whole is greater than the parts. Being a "Double Energy" twin by myself just wouldn't work! My parents, Irwin and Devra Zucker, have always been an inspiration to me. My father taught me that "it doesn't cost anything to be nice, and those who give have all things!" My mother, Devra, has taught me that "too much of a good thing can be wonderful, and you better get while the getting is good." A heartfelt thanks to my "other mother," Marilyn, for teaching me that even through adversity one can stay positive and live life to its fullest! My twin sons, Max and Miles, are fine young men who have so much confidence in themselves. They have taught me how to appreciate their music and style. My daughter Mattea is a beautiful girl who shines her light on everyone she meets. Mattea helped me realize how much I needed a daughter. I have to acknowledge my very funny and loving husband, Daniel, whose wicked sense of humor keeps me smiling. Daniel has taught me to be efficient in life so I have enough energy for him at night!

Thanks to our friends Richard and Claudia Handin for reading over the manuscript and giving wonderful suggestions at our numerous lunch dates. We want to thank friends Kim King Fernandez, Lucia Engel, Samantha Keeping, Athena Hawker, Donna Long, Jill Black, Barbara Berkowitz, Cristina Gavin, Sara Oberman, and Vivianne Gladden for their encouragement.

Thanks to Medeighnia Lentz Photography and Kenji Photography, who kept telling us we looked good. Thanks to our web designer, Angela Stark. Thanks to Armand for his tech support. Thanks to Melinda Angel for sharing her knowledge of nutrition. Thanks to our literary agent, Judith Riven, for being helpful, kind and brilliant. Thanks to Judith Kern for her editorial assistance. Thanks to Cheryl Redmond for editing our book, and giving informative, current and excellent suggestions. Thanks to The Book Publishing Company and their terrific staff, including Kathleen Rosemary, and Cynthia and Bob Holzapfel who share a sincere commitment to publishing creative and wonderful books about health and nutrition. Cynthia, you are a visionary and a genius!

ABOUT THE AUTHORS

Judi and Shari Zucker enjoy a well-deserved reputation as the "Double Energy Twins." They began as cookbook writers while they were teenagers at Beverly Hills High School, where their nutritious lifestyle helped them break the women's one- and two-mile track records. Enthusiastic about sharing their energy secrets, they published *How to Survive Snack Attacks ... Naturally* when they were just seventeen. They are also the authors of *How to Eat Without Meat ... Naturally* and *Double Your Energy with Half the Effort.*

The Zuckers continued their study of health and nutrition at The University of California, Santa Barbara, where they graduated with honors in ergonomics, the combined study of human physiology, physical education, and nutrition. They then served as media specialists for General Mills, publicizing the company's Nature Valley Granola products.

Judi and Shari enjoy successful careers in real estate and interior design, as well as creating and compiling recipes for nutritious low-fat, high-fiber meals. They appear on national and local television talk shows, have taught natural foods cooking classes to adults and children, and maintain their own fitness by running, swimming, and walking daily.

Shari lives with her husband, Daniel Kilstofte, twin sons Max and Miles, and daughter Mattea, and Judi lives with husband Chris Mjelde, daughter Taryn, and son Tanner in southern California.

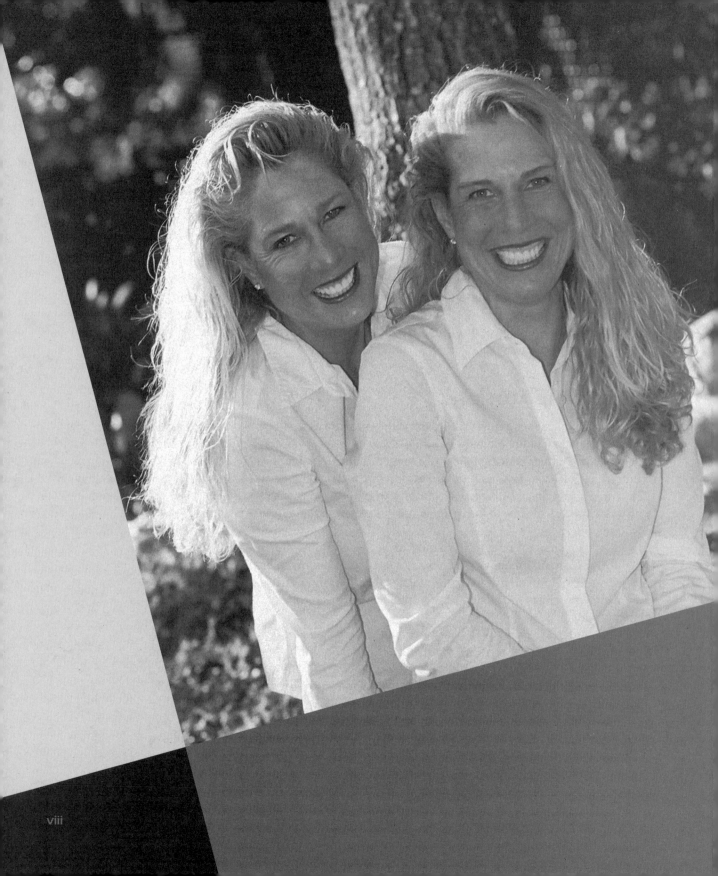

Living It Up!

ON THE DOUBLE ENERGY DIET

We grew up in Beverly Hills, California. Yes, movie stars, palatial estates, and unfortunately, a ton of smog. To get away from the polluted air, our family found refuge in Santa Barbara. We were always taken aback by its beauty. We attended college at the University of California Santa Barbara, and majored in ergonomics, the study of nutrition and physical education.

Santa Barbara is an oasis for the health-conscious. Year round the climate is ideal. It's easy to exercise and eat healthfully here. The area's beauty and invigorating climate persuaded us to stay in Santa Barbara and make it our home. The Double Energy Diet reflects our city's energetic lifestyle and will benefit everyone everywhere.

We became vegetarians (specifically, lacto-ovo vegetarians, a label we'll explain in chapter 1) at eleven years old, when an art teacher convinced us that a meatless diet could increase our energy and improve our performance in track and field. By the time we were in high school we were proficient cooks and voracious eaters of whole, unprocessed "real" foods. In fact, we had already published our first book, *How to Survive Snack Attacks . . . Naturally* (Woodbridge Press 1979), and we were developing plans for our next health-oriented cookbook, *How to Eat Without Meat . . . Naturally* (Woodbridge Press 1981). Plus, we had become addicted to regular aerobic exercise, which conditioned our hearts and lungs and made our energy levels soar!

After earning our college degrees, we decided it was time to put our knowledge of nutrition and exercise to work. We gathered our favorite original recipes—ones that best complemented our active lifestyle—and taught natural foods cooking classes at the local YMCA and area elementary schools. We found that most people are too busy to spend much time in the kitchen. Like you, they work or chase children around, and then spend evenings and weekends enjoying sports, outings, or cultural events. Yet they do want delicious and nutritious meals. Our classes helped us spread the good word that eating for added energy does not require a lot of time, effort, or money. Our diet is unique in its simplicity—and in its freedom from gimmicks. Many of our easy-to-make, nutritionally balanced recipes can stand alone or serve as the heart of a meal.

We advocate a daily meal pattern that can make a tremendous difference in helping you lose fat, pounds, and inches, and easily keep extra pounds from sneaking back on. This pattern, which consists of a light breakfast, moderate lunch, and light dinner, takes into account the fact that most of us feel much too tired to fix a large meal at the end of a long day. You'll find our discussion of this light-moderate-light eating plan (also called the LML Plan) in chapter 3.

The Double Energy Diet doesn't stop with its light-moderate-light approach to eating. Unlike many weight reducing programs, this diet helps you lose weight gradually and permanently while simultaneously boosting your energy with life-enhancing natural foods. It meshes with your busy lifestyle because the recipes do not require much preparation time or large numbers of unusual ingredients. Instead, the diet features contemporary combinations of time-honored, traditional foods, and stresses the indisputable importance of aerobic exercise. Based on sound nutritional and medical information, the Double Energy Diet will awaken your taste buds to the sensational flavors of natural foods—and allow you to satisfy your appetite completely. It will help you arrive at a whole new way of choosing and eating foods

The Double Energy Diet is a lifestyle. We are living proof that it works—we have been living this lifestyle for over thirty years! We have always believed in preventive medicine. We have never been gravely sick, obese or experienced a health crisis that made us all of a sudden "get healthy." We never have to "diet" before a special event such as a wedding or class reunion. We never starve ourselves for weeks to fit into an outfit for a special occasion. Why put yourself through that torture? Plus, those quick weight loss diets don't work; often, you lose weight only to gain more weight once you go off the diet. The difference between the Double Energy Diet and the current diet trends is that the Double Energy Diet works for a lifetime.

We want to share with you why certain diets many not be as effective as you might think. High protein/low carbohydrate diets emphasize meats and seafood and discourage eating carbohydrates. Some carbohydrates, known as simple carbohydrates ("the white stuff"), should be discouraged. Simple carbohydrates include the sugars that are added to food products such as refined breads, pasta, baked goods, juices, flavored milk, and candies. These additives are mostly void of fiber and beneficial nutrients. Foods with a high sugar content and no fiber get digested quickly and are rapidly converted into glucose, which hikes up blood sugar. This forces your pancreas to produce excess insulin to help your body process all the glucose. As a result, your blood sugar takes a huge drop, which sends the "hungry" signal to your brain, triggering you to eat readily available foods to restore your blood sugar quickly. Insulin also prevents the breakdown of stored fats, so the more your insulin levels go up, the more fat you eventually accumulate and the greater your risk for obesity, diabetes, and heart disease. Eliminating sugar from your diet will help fix the elevated blood sugar problem. Sugar depletes the body of B vitamins and robs calcium from hair, blood, bones, and teeth. Sugar ferments in the stomach, stopping secretion of gastric juices and inhibiting the stomach's ability to digest foods. Sugar retards the growth of valuable intestinal bacteria. We believe sugary, refined foods are empty calories—we call them "downer" foods and discuss them further in chapter 2. For now, just remember, "white isn't right"—foods like white bread, white rice, white sugar, and other simple carbohydrates are empty calories.

Unfortunately, high-protein diets also discourage the consumption of complex carbohydrates. Before you set your sights on this type of diet, please keep in mind that complex carbohydrates are important for staying healthy. By complex carbohydrates, we mean unrefined plant foods that contain fiber as well as sugar and starch. Complex carbohydrates are rich in the vitamins, minerals, fiber, and phytochemicals that help fight disease. Carbohydrates provide the body with its main source of energy. The lack of fiber in high-protein diets can cause a sluggish digestive system, which in turn makes you feel tired and bloated. Some people who go on high-protein diets feel weak and unsatiated. Because the brain relies on glucose, supplied by carbohydrates, a low-carbohydrate diet may cause difficulty in concentrating and lack of mental sharpness.

The protein sources in these diets are meat and fish. Eighty percent of the livestock and poultry in the United States are treated with drugs. Ninety percent of the pesticides Americans consume come from meats and dairy instead of vegetables and fruits. Unfortunately, polluted waters have affected marine life, too. High levels of polychlorinated biphenyls (PCBs) and mercury in fish jeopardize our health.

The Zone Diet (which we refer to as the "Hollywood diet," because many actors enjoy this diet) is based on portion sizes and is not very practical. It claims that by combining protein and carbohydrates in a precise way, one can place oneself into a metabolic "zone" where fat loss becomes automatic. As with most high-protein diets, the Zone Diet places too much emphasis on animal protein. The Zone Diet discourages eating products made with wheat and other gluten-containing grains, which it claims can cause bloating. It's true that some people are allergic to wheat and gluten. Allergies can deplete your energy; if you suspect you are allergic, you may want to get a blood test to confirm this. But for most of us, whole grains are valuable sources of vitamins, minerals, and fiber. Weight Watchers and other diet organizations stress calorie counting and use premade meals to help people lose weight. The problem is that these meals are often filled with additives and processed foods. There are more than three hundred chemical additives being used in our foods today. Rule of thumb— if you can't pronounce the ingredient on the label, then it's probably not very healthy to eat. Diets such as Fit For Life, which emphasizes raw fruits and vegetables, Marylu Henner's diet of fresh fruits, vegetables, grains and no meat or dairy products, and the

Pritikin Diet, which emphasizes a low fat diet and rigorous exercise, are better choices for people to follow than high-protein meat-based diets.

We could go on and on dissecting various diets, but the truth is that diet is a lifestyle. Consistency is essential to success. Dr. Phil McGraw, author and television personality, encourages dieters to write a food journal of what they are eating and evaluate their food consumption. Behavior strategies towards food are key in Dr. Phil's philosophy. There is no doubt that mental attitude plays an important role in dieting. You have to want to be healthy and then it is easy to stay healthy.

Every BODY talks; just listen. We are all born with the ability to know when we are hungry and when we are full. Unfortunately, people don't listen to their bodies and they overeat. Years of overeating are equivalent to "body abuse." Fortunately, it's never too late to rejuvenate and get in tune with your body. This book can change your life and double your energy forever!

Get a Jump-Start

WHY THE DOUBLE ENERGY DIET IS FOR YOU

Curiosity has gotten the better of you. As your fingers page tentatively through this volume, your eyes search skeptically for pat formulas and ambiguous promises hidden somewhere in the text. You suspect that you have your hands on yet another fad diet, and you believe that our "dietetic" recipes will ask you to ingest palm fronds, sea urchins, or piles of avocados simply so that you can savor the flavors of our wonderful city, Santa Barbara.

And who ever heard of a diet that can double your energy? All the diets you have tried have only made you feel tired and hungry. Maybe you ended up weighing more than you did when you began the diet.

When you skim through the chapters and examine the recipes in this book, you will discover that we use the term "diet" in its original sense; after all, the word simply refers to whatever each of us eats every day. Like many of today's nutritionists and health-care advisors, we want to encourage a way of eating that you can follow for the rest of your life—not just for a week or a month.

In this book we do just that; we propose a way of eating that will do the following:

- Satisfy your physical hunger as well as your psychological need for chewy, crunchy, smooth, tangy or sweet foods
- Fulfill all your nutritional needs
- Eliminate your need to count calories or carbohydrates
- Drastically reduce the amount of fat in your meals

- Significantly lower your intake of concentrated amounts of pesticides and other food contaminants
- Save you time in the kitchen
- Reduce your food costs
- Help conserve some of the world's energy resources
- Boost your body's energy to new heights

If you want to succeed at this energy program, you will need to choose your foods wisely, exercise, and allow your body time to adjust to the changes you're instigating. However, you'll be able to eat an array of whole, nutritious foods that are rich in fiber and are filling. You will feel satisfied after your meals. You won't need to count calories or carbohydrates, just eat when you are hungry and eat until you feel full. The key is to listen to your body and get in tune with yourself. Moderation will become second nature once you re-educate your taste buds to appreciate the glories of grains, legumes, fruits and vegetables.

No doubt you'll quickly discover that this plan for doubling your energy is exceptionally easy to follow and that foods you crave are simple and quick to prepare. In fact, most of the recipes in this book can stand by themselves as light or moderate meals, accompanied simply by whole-grain bread, cooked grains, or a fresh fruit or vegetable. With little effort, you can make permanent changes in your lifestyle. Even exercise will become an addictive activity for you, and you will enjoy more energy than you've ever had before.

What do we mean by "energy?" Simply defined, energy is an inherent capacity for work, for vigorous activity. The word also denotes the resources (the fuel) used to produce energy in such forms as heat, motion and electricity. Human energy—our ability to sustain ourselves and to move—comes from the energy supplied by elements in food, water, and air. We're sure you're quite familiar with the word "calorie," but did you know that it measures energy? A calorie is not some magical expression of the weight-building capacity of foods; it is the amount of heat energy you need to raise the temperature of one gram of water one degree centigrade, and it's what scientists use to describe the energy value of foods.

How does the Double Energy Diet supply your body with extra energy? The answer is very straightforward: The diet is based on complex carbohydrates, which are essential nutrients found in plant foods. The diet incorporates these complex carbohydrates into our light-moderate-light eating plan, and teaches you how to have a positive attitude towards food and exercise so you'll have more energy than you ever dreamed of! As you'll see in the next chapter, complex carbohydrates are the nutrients that supply our systems with the best and most readily available energy. According to Harold McGee's authoritative kitchen reference, *On Food and Cooking* (Scribner 1984), our bodies find "carbohydrates ... the preferred energy source, the first to be tapped, and when adequately supplied, they spare both fats and proteins from being consumed." Complex carbohydrates supply energy that the body can use efficiently and evenly over time, and they also come packaged with essential amino acids, the building blocks of protein, which are essential to our body's growth.

Because foods derived from plants are so beneficial, and because they have been staples in so many cultures for so many centuries, we have designed our recipes and menus to be essentially lacto-ovo vegetarian. In other words, the Double Energy Diet is centered on plant foods, with limited amounts of dairy products, which add variety and protein and provide necessary minerals and vitamins, including riboflavin, calcium and vitamins A, B_{12}, and D.

If you are a vegan, you'll find it very easy to make all our recipes with nondairy alternatives to milk and cheese. If you are a meat eater who isn't sure whether you want to embark upon a vegetarian regimen, simply try cutting back on the amount of meat you eat. You will feel better. Americans eat too much animal protein, and because that protein usually comes bundled with saturated fats and potentially high levels of contaminants like pesticides and antibiotics, meat consumption contributes to atherosclerosis (blockage of arteries and thickening of artery walls), heart disease, cancer, and other serious illnesses. (See Chapter 2 for a comprehensive look at the problems inherent in animal protein.) If you can reduce the amount of meat in your diet, you will notice that your palate will change, and you may find it quite easy to eliminate meats from your diet entirely. There are plenty of vegetarian alternatives to traditional meat meals, including excellent low-fat, soy- and nut-based products. Companies such as Amy's, Cedarlane, Health is Wealth, and Yves are wonderful. Their products include vegetarian hot dogs, burgers, deli slices, and much more. We recommend taking a walk through the natural foods section of your grocery store or, better yet, shop at your local natural foods store to get acquainted with all the great healthy foods available to you.

Once you accustom your taste buds to the wonderful flavors of whole, unprocessed foods, the ingredients fundamental to our recipes will become staples in your kitchen and your diet. And because you can eat a much higher volume of these complex-carbohydrate foods than animal foods for the same number of calories, you will find that you can satisfy your appetite without worrying about calorie counts. This diet is naturally low in fat, and medical researchers have shown that diets that focus on decreasing fat rather than decreasing calories allow individuals to lose weight spontaneously and to maintain near-ideal weights. Plus those individuals can eat as much as they like of delicious, low-fat foods.

Further, the Double Energy Diet proposes a way of eating that is economical for you and for the world. Grains, legumes, fruits, and vegetables cost very little compared to meats, and less energy is required to get them from the field to your table. According to Frances Moore Lappé's revolutionary book *Diet for A Small Planet* (Ballantine Books 1985), a rancher requires sixteen pounds of grain and soybeans to produce just one pound of beef. Just think how many mouths those sixteen pounds of grain would feed! A meal of grain and soybeans supplies much more usable protein than you can find in one pound of meat, and these plant foods contain no saturated fat or cholesterol.

So not only will following a whole-foods diet increase your personal energy, it will preserve some of the world's energy resources. In a sense it is a transforming diet, an eating plan that is life-preserving. As Lappé notes so eloquently, "what we eat is within our control, yet the act ties us to the economic, political, and ecological order of our whole planet. Even an apparently small change—consciously choosing a diet that is good both for our bodies and for the earth—can lead to a series of choices that transform our whole lives."

Such a diet can transform our future, too; as you'll read in chapter 3, medical researchers have amassed much evidence that too much fat in the diet creates a high risk of colon cancer, breast cancer, atherosclerosis, heart disease, gallstones, and other major health problems. Certain fruits and vegetables, including citrus fruits, cabbage, cauliflower, broccoli, spinach, legumes, and seeds, may actually help prevent cancer by encouraging the body's production of certain enzymes. Plus, the antioxidants found in fresh fruits and vegetables help build the body's immune system against cancer. For this book, we have put together nutritious and delicious energizing recipes, which include life-sustaining plant foods, ones that actually revitalize and prolong your life.

Rev Up Your Body's Engine With Fuel Food

SHIFT TO "UPPER" FOODS

To appreciate the simplicity of the Double Energy Diet, you need to at least survey the complex chemistry of all the foods available to us. Many medical researchers and dieticians have spent lifetimes exploring the intricacies of nutrients and energy balances in humans.

Because we like to keep nutritional information intelligible, we refer to those foods which our bodies convert efficiently to useable energy and which supply important nutrients as "uppers." These are foods at the heart of the Double Energy Diet. At the other end of the food spectrum are "downers," energy sources that transform easily into detrimental body fat, contribute to risk for disease, or carry little nutritional value. To clarify what we mean by "uppers" and "downers" we need to discuss the chemical compounds that distinguish the three main types of nutrients that fuel our bodies: proteins, fats and carbohydrates. Because each serves a necessary function, we cannot label any of these energy sources as strictly an "upper" or a "downer"—each can be either, depending upon a number of criteria.

Protein

Protein is essential to your body's ability to create tissues, to make disease-fighting antibodies, to regulate acidity and alkalinity levels, to move nutrients and oxygen in and out of cells throughout your body, and to help prevent blood clots. Although protein exists in every cell of our bodies, we must replenish our protein supply daily because the human body simply cannot store this invaluable fuel and because a protein deficiency can cause muscle loss. The protein our bodies need for all of the

9

above functions comes from food protein, which consists of many different amino acids. The human body takes apart these dietary amino acids and creates new ones. However, of the twenty-two amino acids humans need to survive, eight must be supplied directly from food because our bodies cannot manufacture them. These eight essential amino acids, all of which must be present in our systems simultaneously, are isoleucine, leucine, lysine, methionine, threonine, valine, phenylalanine, and tryptophan. In addition, the amino acid histidine is essential to children's growth.

When the essential amino acids are present together in a food, nutritionists say that the food supplies complete protein; in other words, that food by itself will meet all your protein needs. All foods that come from animals (meats, eggs, milk products—every animal-supplied food except gelatin) furnish your body with complete protein. Because most plant foods are incomplete proteins—that is, they don't supply sufficient amounts of all the essential amino acids—in the past it was believed that plant foods had to be carefully combined in the same meal in order to provide "complementary" protein combinations. In fact, you can get complete protein by eating a variety of vegetarian foods over the course of a day, because complementary proteins do not need to be consumed at the same meal. *The New Becoming Vegetarian* by Vesanto Melina and Brenda Davis (Healthy Living Publications 2003) gives excellent examples of how eating a plant-based diet throughout the day gives you "complete protein." This book is an excellent guide to a healthy and practical vegetarian diet for all ages, and shows how even strict vegetarians (vegans) who eat nothing other than plant-based foods can get adequate protein from whole grains, nuts and legumes.

What turns animal-based foods into "downer" foods? Although many people believe the only way they are going to get enough protein is through animal-based foods, ironically, many of these foods provide more fat than protein. Many meats and cheeses have undesirable levels of saturated fat, and offer absolutely no fiber.

Indeed, as researchers point out repeatedly, we Americans consume far more protein—particularly animal protein—than we can ever possibly use. Only about 10 to 15 percent of the adult male's diet needs to consist of protein. Of that protein, only 20 percent needs to be complete. Our bodies use protein for energy only after we burn fats and carbohydrates. Excess protein simply converts to fat, something few of us need more of. Too much protein also prompts the body to lose bone-building calcium, contributes to high blood pressure, and can eventually damage the kidneys because they cannot process all the extra nitrogen that is intrinsic to protein.

Furthermore, scientists have found increasing evidence that red meat and poultry contain dangerous, concentrated levels of contaminants, such as the pesticides applied to the grains that animals eat in such great quantities. The meat Americans eat may also contain residues of the antibiotics and hormones that ranchers use to prevent disease and to promote growth in livestock. Even fish, which offer beneficial unsaturated fats, are potential sources of food poisoning because of the toxic microorganisms the fish have consumed. Fish may also contain dangerous chemical contaminants like DDT or polychlorinated biphenyls (PCBs). Consumption of chemicals harbored in the flesh of livestock, poultry, and fish may lead to serious health problems for humans. High levels of mercury in shark, swordfish, king mackerel and tilefish may harm brain development in unborn babies and young children. Uncooked shellfish can carry hepatitis.

Many people eat fish because fish oil is rich in polyunsaturated fats known as omega-3 fatty acids. We recommend eating flaxseeds or flaxseed oil or taking flaxseed oil capsules instead. These all contain a type of omega-3 fatty acid called alpha-linolenic acid. Omega-3 fatty acids normalize cholesterol and triglyceride levels, suppress inflammation and allergies, alleviate depression, heal dry skin, and combat fatigue. Omega-3 fatty acids have the ability to break down cholesterol in the lining of blood vessels, as well as serving as a solvent for saturated fats in the diet. Less cholesterol in the body and bloodstream reduces the likelihood of heart disease and its complications. It also can lower blood pressures. Like flaxseed oil, evening primrose oil, rich in gamma linolenic acid, is wonderful for the skin and is known to help symptoms of premenstrual syndrome.

Biomagnification is the increased concentration of chemicals, pesticides, and toxins that come from animals that eat grains and vegetables exposed to pesticides. These pesticides concentrate one thousand times more in the animal's fat, and if you eat that animal then you are most likely transporting pesticides, heavy metals, mercury, or lead into your healthy body.

To circumvent such problems, you can acquire all the protein you need from plant foods (preferably organically grown), which possess varying amounts and numbers of the eight essential amino acids. People have flourished for centuries on cuisines that pair complementary plant proteins without understanding the science behind their food choices. The traditional diets of many cultural groups feature very little animal protein, but large amounts of grains and legumes. Good "upper" food combinations, used often in the Double Energy Diet, include whole grains with legumes, nuts with legumes, and seeds with legumes. Enjoy these "upper" food combinations at the same meal or throughout the day. Your body will amass all of the amino acids it needs to function properly. You don't have to worry about getting "enough protein."

The foundation for human diets in many countries for countless centuries, grains include corn, wheat, oats, quinoa, buckwheat, rice, rye, barley, sorghum, amaranth, and millet. Grains can be eaten in their whole form, or in a variety of whole-grain products such as breads, cereals, pastas, crackers, couscous, and tortillas. Extremely high in valuable nutrients, legumes (dried peas and beans) have likewise fueled the forgers of great civilizations. The legume family includes soybeans, peanuts, lentils, chickpeas (garbanzo beans), black beans, various white beans, split peas, kidney beans, lima beans, pinto beans, black-eyed peas, red beans, and more.

Seeds and nuts, powerhouses of protein, complement other plant foods superbly. However, these high-energy foods also contain plenty of fat (though mostly unsaturated) and calories, so eat them sparingly and choose either raw or dry-roasted unsalted varieties. Technically speaking, seeds come from the fruits of plants and contain the embryos for the next generation of their species; good choices include pumpkin and squash seeds, sesame seeds, and sunflower seeds. The dried fruit of trees, edible nuts, include chestnuts, almonds, hazelnuts (filberts), pignoli (pine nuts), pecans, pistachios, and walnuts. Macadamia nuts and coconut offer less nutrition than other nuts and seeds; they contain little protein and lots of saturated fat, and that's probably why they taste so good!

As we mentioned earlier, dairy products and eggs provide complete protein in themselves. Further, their protein power multiplies when you combine them with plant foods. When shopping for dairy products and eggs, buy organic when possible. Look for milk that doesn't contain bovine growth hormone (rBGH). Bovine growth hormone may cause an increased risk of cancer and diabetes. Organic milk is free of this hormone. Antibiotics are injected in most hens. Look for eggs that come from cage-free (free-range) hens that are fed vegetarian diets.

We don't eat lots of dairy products because we don't digest milk well. Instead we drink rice milk. We have no problem digesting cultured dairy products such as plain yogurt and cottage cheese. Natural plain nonfat yogurt is rich in protein, calcium, vitamin B_{12}, zinc, selenium, magnesium, riboflavin, and probiotics (bacteria that are beneficial for your digestive system). Cottage cheese is a good protein source filled with calcium and B vitamins, and some brands contain probiotics as well.

Fats

As we mentioned earlier, protein that comes from animals often travels with large quantities of dietary fat. A potential "downer" food, fat contains nine calories per gram—more than twice as many as proteins or carbohydrates (which each contain four calories per gram). Fat provides few nutrients, and it poses serious health risks to those whose daily intake exceeds 30 percent of their total calories. And it's easy to eat too much fat because you must eat more to feel full and because fat tastes so good to most of us.

You may be surprised to learn how little fat you need to eat in order to manufacture the fat your body needs to survive. Body fat insulates and cushions your organs and provides oils for your hair and skin. If you are a woman, you need fat to help build prostaglandins, the chemicals that regulate your sex hormones. Nonetheless, each of us only needs to consume one tablespoon of fat per day to maintain good nutrition. Our bodies use proteins and carbohydrates to manufacture body fat for calorie storage, and our systems only need that one tablespoon of polyunsaturated fat from a vegetable source in order to obtain the essential chemical called linoleic acid, which we need to create body fat. That one tablespoon of polyunsaturated fat also helps our digestive system absorb the fat soluble vitamins A, D, E, and K. However, our bodies need absolutely no saturated fat—the kind that comes from animal foods. What do the terms polyunsaturated and saturated mean? You have probably heard the word polyunsaturated applied to the cooking oils you buy at your supermarket. Really, there are three kinds of fats—those that contain primarily saturated, polyunsaturated, and monounsaturated fatty acids.

Saturated fats, the "downer" fats that pose the greatest danger to our health, occur in animal tissues and in the coconut oil, palm oil, and cocoa butter so frequently used in candies and processed foods. For those interested in the technical side of things, these fats acquired their name because the fatty acids, composed of carbon and hydrogen atoms, that make up saturated fats have no double or triple bonds and no more room for any additional hydrogen—in other words, the molecules are completely full or "saturated." Solid at room temperature, saturated fats are easy to recognize. Butter, lard, chicken fat, and all the marbling in "high-quality" meats are saturated fats that researchers link to cancers of the colon, breast, uterus, ovaries, and other parts of the body. Plus saturated fats clog circulatory systems and cause heart disease. Cholesterol is not the same thing as saturated fat; it is a lipid molecule found in all animals, including those with little or no saturated fat, like shellfish. However, saturated fat and cholesterol often travel hand in hand, and saturated fat provokes your body's own cholesterol-manufacturing machine.

Humans need cholesterol to make cell membranes and certain hormones, and to form vitamin D molecules. We also need this vital substance to produce bile salts that help the intestine metabolize dietary fats. However, after the age of six months, our bodies can synthesize—in the liver, intestines, and elsewhere—all the cholesterol we need without the assistance of additional dietary cholesterol. Although eating foods that contain cholesterol decreases the amount of cholesterol produced by the liver, the synthesis of cholesterol continues to some extent in other tissues. In addition, some studies indicate that dietary cholesterol may not be used in the same way in which our naturally synthesized cholesterol is used; in fact dietary cholesterol may go almost directly to the blood vessels. Thus we end up with far more cholesterol in our bodies than we need. Indeed, we have difficulty getting rid of excess cholesterol that accumulates in our bodies and becomes deposited in our blood vessels. Scientists now believe that physical inactivity and emotional stress also increase the amount of cholesterol in our blood. We are firm believers that stress not only can elevate cholesterol levels in people, but can contribute to many other diseases.

To complicate matters further, our bodies possess what mass-media health literature calls "good" cholesterol and "bad" cholesterol. You see, cholesterol gets around in the blood by means of complex substances that are both fat (lipid) and protein. These cholesterol-carrying lipoproteins come in three main varieties: high-density lipoproteins (HDLs), low-density lipoproteins (LDLs) and very-low-density lipoproteins (VLDLs). In general, medical scientists refer colloquially to the HDLs as "good" because they take cholesterol away from the artery walls and transport it to the liver, where the HDLs also help to eliminate excess cholesterol. For these reasons, HDLs, which are the primary vehicles by which fats derived from plant foods travel, seem to prevent heart and artery disease. Aerobic exercise seems to increase the levels of HDL-transported cholesterol.

On the other hand, LDLs and VLDLs, low-density and very-low-density lipoproteins, arise in the liver when the diet contains lots of saturated fats, and they tend to keep cholesterol in circulation. They deliver cholesterol to cells that need it, but they fail to remove excess cholesterol from artery walls. Most of the cholesterol in our bodies travels inside LDLs and VLDLs, the notoriously "bad" kind of cholesterol carrier.

Polyunsaturated fats, which are those supplied by plant foods, travel primarily via HDLs, which reduce the amount of cholesterol in your blood and may help to lower blood pressure. These fats acquired their name ("poly" means "many") because their fatty acid molecules contain more than one double or triple bond between hydrogen and carbon clusters and can accept at least four more hydrogen atoms. Polyunsaturated fats occur as oils and remain liquid at room temperature: oils rich in these fats include soybean, safflower, sunflower, corn, and linseed or flaxseed (which, like fish, contains valuable omega-3 fatty acids). Walnuts are also a good source of polyunsaturated fats. Sources of monounsaturated fats, whose fatty acid molecules have just one double bond and can accept just two more hydrogen atoms, include olive oil, peanut oil, avocados, and most nuts. These fats may be even more effective in reducing cholesterol in our blood than polyunsaturated oils.

Although monounsaturated and polyunsaturated oils qualify as "upper" foods when used sparingly, they can be problematic for our bodies if food manufacturers have hydrogenated them. Hydrogenation is a process by which polyunsaturated or monounsaturated oil is made more saturated, as in the case of many margarines and vegetable shortenings. According to some studies, hydrogenated oils may allow cancer-causing chemicals easier access to certain cells. We recommend buying non-hydrogenated margarine made from expeller-pressed oil.

When selecting a cooking fat, simply remember that too much of any kind of fat increases body weight, and studies are beginning to indicate that large amounts of even the unsaturated fats may contribute to the development of cancer and of gallstones. Plus, unknown to you, your body may be genetically predisposed to produce far more "bad" cholesterol than "good" cholesterol—no matter which kind of fat you eat. For these reasons, we have designed the Double Energy Diet, an eating plan high in complex carbohydrates, to limit the amount of fat you consume to 30 percent or less of your total calorie intake.

Carbohydrates

Increasing your consumption of whole foods that contain complex carbohydrates and fiber will quite naturally lead to a decrease in dietary fat because complex-carbohydrate foods usually contain little fat—and no deadly saturated fat—and because such foods fill you up without filling you with calories. Contrary to popular belief, most "natural" carbohydrates are not fattening at all! They are the "upper" foods you combine to create complete, useable proteins. (See the section on protein above.) What's more, complex carbohydrates are an incredible source of efficiently burned energy.

Complex carbohydrates are one of two major types of carbohydrates, which are organic compounds composed of carbon, hydrogen, and oxygen. The complex types are starches that consist of long chains of sugar molecules, which our bodies break down gradually, thus releasing energy incrementally. The grains, legumes, vegetables, fruits, seeds, and nuts we discussed in the above section on complementary proteins are complex-carbohydrate foods.

The other type of carbohydrates are simple carbohydrates, composed of just one or two molecules of sugar. These simple sugars include fructose, glucose, and sucrose, or table sugar.

Plants make both simple and complex carbohydrates during photosynthesis, the process by which water, carbon dioxide, and sunlight become chemical energy. Milk, which contains the sugar lactose, is the only food from an animal source that possesses a carbohydrate in any significant amount.

Once we eat any kind of carbohydrate, our bodies break it down into glucose, which circulates through the body and supplies the cells with their favorite kind of fuel. Interestingly, the brain and other tissues in the nervous system can use only glucose for energy: fats simply won't do. Our bodies can store only about one half of a day's supply of glucose as glycogen in the liver and muscles, and we will begin to convert (inefficiently and sometimes dangerously) body protein and fat into glucose if our glycogen supply runs short. If we must rely on protein or fat for our glucose, then we overtax our kidneys and can cause our bodies serious harm. Humans cannot function properly without the right glucose levels; if our metabolism of the substance goes awry, we end up with diabetes or hypoglycemia.

If all of the carbohydrates we eat end up as glucose, why does the Double Energy Diet revolve around complex rather than simple carbohydrates? Aren't all carbohydrates the same in the end? And aren't straight sugars better sources of quick energy than complex carbohydrates? Sure, but therein lies the problem: the energy from simple carbohydrates is much too quickly enjoyed. Not only do the sugars in candy bars, soft drinks, or table sugar rot your teeth, they also cause a sugar "high" that is followed rapidly by a crash in blood sugar. These "downer" foods trigger excessive bursts of insulin, the hormone that regulates blood sugar levels, which rapidly takes care of all the sugar in the blood. A sugar "low" can leave you feeling a little depressed and probably even hungrier than you were before. In addition, sugars that don't travel with starches, or complex carbohydrates, provide little in the way of nutrients. Simple carbohydrates are those "empty calories" you've heard so much about. When we use them as substitutes for other foods, simple carbohydrates may prevent us from obtaining the vitamins and minerals we need.

The way that different carbohydrates break down in your body is the basis of the popular glycemic index .The glycemic index, or GI, is a way to measure the effect of a given food on blood sugar levels. Authors of diets such as Atkins, The Zone, South Beach, and Sugar Busters have embraced the concept as a "scientific" formula for losing weight. A high GI rating means that a food is broken down very quickly into glucose, which sets off a chain reaction in the body. Your blood sugar (glucose) spikes up. Your pancreas releases a shot of insulin to drive it down. Your glucose can fall rapidly, at which point the liver starts putting out more glucose and fatty acids to stabilize the situation. Then you will probably feel hungry again or in extreme cases dizzy or tired. Foods with a high GI tend to be refined carbohydrates such as white breads, cakes, and candies—also known as junk food. Lower GI foods are made up of complex carbohydrates that have lots of fiber and nutritional value; these are preferred. Studies have found that people on high-protein diets lost weight faster than people on low-fat diets with a low GI index within a six month period, but by the end of a year the amount of weight lost was equal. While the glycemic index is a useful tool, you don't need GI numbers to know that weight loss and good health simply comes from eating fruits, vegetables, and whole-grain foods and drinking plenty of water.

The complex carbohydrates found in fruits, vegetables, grains, and beans come with wide varieties of nutrients and various forms of fiber, the plant substances (cellulose, hemicellulose, pectin, lignin, gums, mucilage, and polysaccharides) that our human digestive enzymes cannot break down. Dietary fiber makes you feel full and keeps your digestive tract in top shape. In addition, scientific studies show that the dietary fiber in complex carbohydrates acts as a natural laxative and prevents bowel disease, heart disease, and cancers of the colon and breast. Fiber satisfies your psychological need to chew, absorbs water and makes you feel full, interferes with your body's absorption of fats, and indirectly changes the amount of glucose you absorb. Thus a fiber-rich diet may quite naturally reduce the calories, cholesterol, and saturated fats you consume. Fruits, vegetables, and whole grains (which contain bran) are the best sources of dietary fiber.

Fiber-rich complex carbohydrates can supply your body with all the vitamins, minerals, protein, and fat necessary for healthy living. Investigators of traditional diets, such as those of many African and Chinese people, and scientific research suggest that up to 60 percent of your total food energy should come from complex carbohydrates. In addition, complex-carbohydrate whole foods have not been associated in any way with any major disease. And because digestive enzymes break complex carbohydrates into glucose slowly, plant foods cause blood sugar levels to stay pretty even and make energy available for relatively long periods of time . . . and energy is what we're after!

Raw Foods Energize

There is no doubt that eating fresh fruits and vegetables gives you more energy. Fruits and vegetables contain naturally-occurring plant chemicals called phytochemicals. Many phytochemicals serve as antioxidants, capturing free radicals in our bodies and preventing them from damaging our DNA. Antioxidants support the immune system and help reduce the incidence of all cancers. Phytochemicals also lower cholesterol, detoxify the liver, clear up nasal congestion, and heal stomach ulcers.

We are all born with biologically active proteins called enzymes. There are thousands of enzymes present in your body that are essential to all life's processes. Enzymes produce chemical reactions that allow you to breathe, move, and think. Your enzyme supply is depleted when you eat too much fat, protein, and processed sugars. Overcooking or microwaving foods can deplete enzymes in your body, which can cause your pancreas, stomach, and liver to overproduce enzymes to balance your body's needs. This creates an enzyme imbalance, which depletes your body of energy. On the other hand, eating fresh uncooked fruits and vegetables, which also contain enzymes, supports the enzymes in your body. Papaya and pineapple, for example, are enzyme-rich fruits that aid digestion. In order to have optimum energy, your diet should be high in fresh fruit, vegetables, and sprouts.

Other "Uppers" and "Downers"

As you have seen in our discussion above, complex carbohydrates are the primary "upper" food fuels for your body. Some dietary proteins and fats also qualify, but only complex carbohydrates from natural, unprocessed foods supply all the nutrients you need without contributing any negative factors.

Because the lack of certain vitamins and minerals can rob the body of energy, it is often a good idea to support "upper" foods with "upper" supplements. For example, B vitamins support healthy energy, appetite, red blood cell production, and production of hydrochloric acid, which aids digestion. Vitamins A, C, and E, zinc, and the amino acids glycine, serine, taurine, and tyrosine, are also particularly important for energy. Coenzyme Q-10 (known as ubiquinone or CoQ-10) is an essential component of the cellular compartment (known as mitochondria), where it plays a major role in energy production in the body. CoQ-10 is an antioxidant found in high concentrations in the human heart, liver, kidney, spleen, and pancreas. It helps protect your body from free radicals and helps preserve vitamin E, the major antioxidant of cell membranes and blood cholesterol. CoQ-10 is available in vegetarian capsules.

Some people swear by energy-enhancing supplements such as ginseng, spirulina, and royal jelly. Although these supplements may increase your energy, the one we have found to be most worthwhile is rhodiola. Rhodiola, also known as "golden root," is an herb that fights off fatigue. It has been used to decrease fatigue and depression for hundreds of years in traditional Asian medicine. Rhodiola is considered an adaptogen. An adaptogen helps the body to adjust to different stressors, and also helps the body to reassume homeostasis (the balance between various bodily functions and the chemical composition of fluids and tissues) once the stressor is no longer around. Basically, rhodiola can offer generalized, non-specific resistance to physical, chemical, and biological stressors one may experience in everyday life.

More than a million people suffer from chronic fatigue syndrome (CFS), sometimes called chronic fatigue and immune dysfunction syndrome (DFIDS), which causes debilitating fatigue. Besides extreme fatigue this syndrome can include flu-like symptoms, headaches, muscle aches, inability to concentrate, allergies, anxiety, and depression. These symptoms may be brought on by viral infections or stressful events. Taking rhodiola and B vitamins, along with altering one's diet, may dramatically improve even these extreme cases of fatigue.

Another essential "upper" fuel is water, our bodies' most critical nutrient and lubricant. A simple combination of hydrogen and oxygen, water composes about 60 to 70 percent of our body weight and is the main constituent of blood. Water keeps everything in our bodies moving, speeds fat metabolism, and regulates our internal temperature. Dehydration is the number one factor for fatigue. For those of us on a high-carbohydrate, high-fiber diet, water is especially important for keeping our digestion and elimination systems in good working order. Furthermore, water maintains the structure and function of enzymes responsible for breaking down fat. In the absence of pure water, fat metabolism is retarded. Water should be a major component of any weight management program.

In *The Energy Edge* (LifeLine Press 1999), Pamela Smith discusses how our bodies continually lose water throughout the day. Even breathing uses up stored fluids in the body. Every time you exhale, water from your body is carried out with your breath; the amount adds up to about two cups per day. Water also evaporates from your skin to cool your body, even when you aren't aware of sweating. These losses can build up to ten cups per day. When you're perspiring heavily, that amount doubles! Don't rely on your thirst mechanism to let you know you need water because by the time you're thirsty you have already lost a significant amount of fluid. Carry a water bottle with you wherever you go. Consistently drink water all day long in order to sustain your health and energy.

Unfortunately, many of us drink water that contains contaminants, which may interfere with good health. Tap water may even contain suspected carcinogens (cancer-causing elements), like polychlorinated biphenyls (PCBs) and chloroform. Contamination from viruses, bacteria, pesticides, toxic heavy metals, industrial chemicals, asbestos, and simply the additives cities use to treat public water can cause serious medical problems. Some water supplies also contain excessive amounts of sodium. If you drink your water straight from the tap, be sure to have it tested periodically for contaminants. And if the water coming from your faucet ever looks cloudy, boil it for at least ten minutes before using it to cook or drink. You may want to invest in water filters or drink bottled water. For an informative overview of all these water options, take a look at Earl Mindell's extremely helpful book titled *Unsafe at Any Meal* (Warner Books 1987).

While we're speaking about the liquid so essential to our bodies, we should mention several beverages that people imbibe in place of water, but that certainly qualify as "downers" for our metabolisms.

Drinking alcoholic beverages is simply consuming "empty calories." Alcoholic beverages are simple sugars that have no nutrients. People who drink alcohol in excess tend to consume little else and can eventually suffer from malnutrition and dehydration. Not only does alcohol contain no vitamins or minerals, it also draws water out of brain cells and prevents your body from absorbing nutrients from other foods. Because alcohol is also a drug that alters brain functions and acts as an anesthetic, its consumption is the primary cause of almost half our nation's traffic accidents each year. Medical scientists link heavy drinking with liver disease, high blood pressure, stroke, heart disease, cancer, and fetal alcohol syndrome, the terribly sad condition affecting babies of women who drink heavily during their pregnancies. Even a few alcoholic drinks can depress your immune system and increase your susceptibility to infections, and alcohol can react adversely with many medications. In fact, the additives in many alcoholic beverages can cause adverse reactions all by themselves. Need we say more?

Other mind-altering "downer" beverages that need to be eliminated from a sound diet are coffee, tea, cocoa, and colas. These beverages contain caffeine, theophylline and/or theobromine, stimulants that affect the heart, brain, central nervous system, respiratory system, and kidneys. Like alcohol, they dehydrate rather than replenish your body's fluid supply; these stimulants stress the kidneys and act as diuretics. Although caffeine-containing beverages can speed up the rate at which you metabolize fuels, they can also increase your hunger because they stimulate the release of insulin, which clears glucose from your blood. Caffeine-containing drinks may indeed make you more mentally alert for a while, but your body will come to depend on them, and withdrawal from the beverages can result in headaches, depression, fatigue, and nausea. Researchers have linked high caffeine intake with higher incidences of miscarriage among pregnant women as well as high blood pressure and elevated blood cholesterol. Some countries, such as France and Denmark, have banned "energy drinks" like Red Bull because of elevated caffeine levels. One can of Red Bull contains 80 milligrams of caffeine. Coca Cola, chocolate bars, and even Excedrin Pain Reliever all contain caffeine. As you see, caffeine-containing products can sabotage an otherwise nutritious diet and healthy lifestyle, and they can trigger the same sorts of energy crashes that sweets do. Instead of coffee, try decaffeinated green tea or peppermint tea. Green tea contains theanine, a component that has a stress-reducing effect on the brain, and it's high in antioxidants. Peppermint oil is known to increase alertness by stimulating a nerve in the face called the trigeminal nerve.

Colas also pose another problem: like all soft drinks they leach calcium from our systems, interfere with iron absorption, dose our bodies with potentially harmful additives (like brominated vegetable oils and sodium alginate), give us quick energy fixes that end up as energy crashes, provide us with no nutritive value except almost pure calories, and bolster our craving for additional sweets. Even diet soft drinks condition us to crave sugar because the body believes it is consuming huge amounts of sugar and acts accordingly. Diet drinks prevent us from reconditioning our palate to desire fewer sweeteners, and diet beverages contain far too much sodium, another potential "downer."

While alcohol and caffeine cause the loss of valuable fluids, another chemical, salt, or sodium chloride, can cause excessive retention of fluids, resulting in high blood pressure and fatigue. Forty percent of the salt molecule is sodium, the mineral necessary for many of our bodies' functions—and the mineral responsible for such conditions as the hypertension mentioned above and the bloated feeling associated with premenstrual tension. Sodium occurs naturally in plenty of whole, unprocessed foods, and certain vegetables and dairy products (such as celery, spinach, beets, cheeses, and eggs) possess high levels of the mineral. But what concerns dieticians and physicians is the sodium that we add to our foods, either by processing or canning them or simply by passing the salt shaker over perfectly tasty foods. (Examples of highly salted packaged or prepared foods include potato chips, pickles, ready-to-eat cereals, instant puddings, canned vegetables, commercially baked goods, and of course, processed meats, which also contain other dangerous additives.) You will obtain more than enough sodium to regulate the fluids in your membranes if you stick to the recipes in *The Double Energy Diet*, and by weaning yourself from added salt, you can fight fatigue and appreciate the flavors of whole foods even more. Discover the unique culinary personalities of fresh or dried herbs, which make terrific, healthful alternatives to table salt, the ultimate "downer" food additive.

Tobacco is a downer, and smoking may be the Western world's greatest health danger. According to World Health Organization surveys, smoking plays a direct role in more than 500,000 American deaths yearly, including those from cancer, heart disease, respiratory disease, fire, and other accidents. Secondhand smoke (passive smoking or breathing someone else's smoke) is damaging to the lungs, particularly those of children. The Environmental Protection Agency (EPA) has stated that passive smoke is "the most dangerous airborne carcinogen" in the United States. The EPA estimates that up to 5,000 Americans die each year from breathing someone else's cigarette smoke.

If you want to maintain good health, smoking must have no place in your life at all! Not only does smoking cause fatal diseases, it interferes with the absorption of vital nutrients, and causes a significant vitamin C deficit in the blood. Any vitamin deficiency can deplete the body of energy.

Another downer worth mentioning is stress. In *Your Body, Your Diet* (Ballantine Books 2001), Elizabeth Dane states that stress is an inescapable part of daily life that not only gobbles up nutrients but also makes the body retain the minerals that stimulate or excite it while inhibiting the substances that calm and regenerate. Stress changes the body's ability to function efficiently. Stress is energy depleting! When you feel "stressed out," start to breathe. Take a few deep breaths and remind your body to relax. Assure yourself that you will be fine. Start to think "optimally" by asking yourself, how can I make this situation better? Soon you will be able to figure out how to deal with your situation in a calm matter. Proper breathing, eating nutritious foods, drinking water, and exercising can train your body to be "stress ready," and you will successfully glide through stressful situations.

The Eight Greats

We have found that incorporating these eight great energy foods into your diet will give you increased stamina:

1. **Flaxseed**: Flaxseed is a terrific source of fiber and alpha-linolenic acid (a type of omega–3 fatty acid), which serves as an anti-inflammatory agent.

2. **Berries**: Berries are full of fiber and cancer-fighting antioxidants. Blueberries are particularly high in antioxidants.

3. **Nuts**: Most nuts contain monounsaturated fat, which helps lower LDL ("bad") cholesterol, reducing the risk of heart disease. Eating nuts also helps prevent type 2 diabetes. Almonds are especially high in fiber, protein, vitamin E, magnesium, potassium, monounsaturated fat, and flavonoids. Walnuts are high in omega-3 fatty acids.

4. **Sprouts**: Sprouts (like alfalfa, radish, and broccoli sprouts) are filled with antioxidants, protein, and enzymes that aid healthy digestion.

5. **Apples**: Apples are a great source of fiber; one apple has 5 grams, which is 20 percent of the daily recommended amount. Apples are high in pectin, a fiber component that aids digestion and helps reduce the absorption of cholesterol, as well as vitamin A, C, and niacin, and minerals such as phosphorus, iron, and potassium. These flavonoid-filled fruits contain pyruvate, which helps reduce the risk of heart disease. Pyruvate forms in the body when carbohydrates and protein convert into energy. Pyruvate appears to work as a weight loss aid by cranking up the resting metabolic rate, which is the minimum number of calories the body burns. Other fruits that aid digestion include papaya and pineapple.

6. **Water**: Water keeps your body hydrated, moving, and energized.

7. **Oatmeal**: This grain is rich in selenium, zinc, thiamin, phytochemicals and fiber.

8. **Soybeans**: These legumes are a complete protein source, rich in potassium, folate, iron, magnesium, thiamin, fiber, and calcium. Tofu and other soy products are high in vegetable protein and complex carbohydrates that burn slowly, balancing blood sugar levels and sustaining energy for an extended period of time. Natural isoflavones found in soybeans have been shown to function similarly to estrogen replacement therapy to help ease symptoms of menopause.

In summary, we recommend that you ease yourself into the Double Energy Diet by:

- avoiding "downer" foods: meats (which are high in saturated fats and cholesterol), large amounts of any kind of fat, and foods filled with sugar and fat.

- dropping all "downer" beverages—alcohol, caffeine-containing beverages and soft drinks—from your diet.

- training your body to be "stress ready" in order to minimize the energy-depleting effects of stress.
- eating a wide variety of "upper" foods—complex carbohydrates and low-fat or nonfat dairy products—to promote high energy.
- drinking plenty of water (about eight glasses a day) to keep your body operating in high gear.

The LML Plan

THE OPTIMAL ENERGY EATING PATTERN

Now that you have a grasp of the kinds of foods that will spur your energy, you need to think about the times of day at which you'll eat those vitalizing foods. When you eat is almost as important as what you eat. As we've said before, you will eventually retrain your taste buds and your metabolism so that you can pretty much eat as much as you want of what we call "upper" foods. However, you will find that your body will maintain peak energy levels if you plan your meals to accommodate your body's natural rhythms—if you eat a light breakfast, a moderate lunch, and a light dinner (we refer to it as the LML Plan). A meal pattern that's unique to the Double Energy Diet in that it contradicts contemporary practices as well as most other diets' recommendations, this plan nonetheless reflects the traditional eating patterns of other cultures.

Delaying or omitting any meal may make you feel cranky and fatigued: hunger can even cause symptoms like headaches and dizziness. On the other hand, eating gobs of food when your body doesn't need much or eating late at night when you can't burn calories effectively can bring on bulges where you don't want them.

Amazingly, healthy bodies have an innate knowledge about when and how much to eat. Sure, certain areas of your mind often override the brain's own intuitive sense of what's right for the stomach, especially when you're not in reasonable physical shape at the moment. But you can learn how to tune in to the wisdom of your own body—how to pay attention to the signals emitted by the parts of the brain that regulate hunger and thirst. And you can become aware of your circadian rhythms. What do we mean by circadian rhythms? They're the biological rhythms that govern the inner workings of humans, the ones that tend to synchronize with what's going on in our environments but that don't depend on anything external to us. A chronobiologist (a scientist who studies time cycles in the natural world) named Franz Halberg first introduced the term while conducting experiments in Minneapolis in 1959; Halberg used it to describe biological rhythms that have a period of about 24 hours (*circa diem*, Latin for "about a day"). As Jeremy Campbell explains in *Winston Churchill's Afternoon Nap* (Simon & Schuster 1986), a terrifically readable book on the human experience of time, "the body knows what time of day or night it is, and so prepares itself for waking or sleeping, feeding and fasting. The changes going on inside the body keep a step ahead of the changes going on outside. This is a strategy for survival in business."

Over the past few decades, chronobiologists have discovered innumerable patterns in the internal mechanisms that govern our appetite, temperature, blood pressure, cell division, hormone production, digestion, and every other process in our bodies. We have certain metabolic rhythms that govern how our bodies use calories, and we burn carbohydrates more effectively in the morning than we do at night. A given meal eaten every morning for a week may result in weight loss, while the identical meal eaten every evening for a week may cause weight gain. Studies show that the body uses dietary fuel differently at different times of the day.

Although your body processes carbohydrates better in the earlier part of the day, it's important not to break a night's fast with a food overload. Too big a breakfast will make anyone feel sluggish and unable to take advantage of the peak intellectual capacity that occurs during the morning hours. However, no breakfast at all may be even more disastrous for your body. As renowned cardiologist Michael DeBakey affirms, failure to break the night's fast will make your blood sugar levels crash, causing weakness, lethargy, concentration difficulties, headaches, or even nausea spells. Plus, you will wind up overeating later in the day. For all of the above reasons, the Double Energy Diet includes plenty of recipes that make nutritious, quick-to-fix, light breakfasts that tell the taste buds (and the rest of the body) to rise and shine.

The body handles food well at midday, and it needs slowly released energy to maintain performance over the afternoon. Deepak Chopra, in his book *Boundless Energy* (Harmony Books 1995), notes that eating one's main meal of the day at lunch time, rather than in the evening, works with the body's internal biological rhythms. These rhythms are of the natural world around us, and therefore the digestive fire is brightest at the same time that the sun is highest in the sky. Hence, digestion is sharpest at noontime.

Of course, there is always the danger of sleepiness after a full lunch, but most people experience some sleepiness in the early afternoon regardless of what they've eaten. According to some scientists, this tendency is probably built into our systems: our ancestors slept during the middle of the day to avoid the hot sun. Our neighbors in Mexico and in Mediterranean and South American countries probably have the right idea: they pay attention to their circadian rhythms and enjoy rejuvenating siestas (naps) after their large midday meals. And take a look at little children; they often nap quite comfortably after their noon munch. Unfortunately, the American workday does not permit such pleasures as afternoon naps; however, a brief walk after lunch will do wonders to keep your brain in good working order and it is a much better choice than having coffee during your "coffee break." Research shows that mental capacity does increase again in a few hours after a high-carbohydrate lunch. If you eat most of your food fuel at lunch, you have plenty of time to burn it off before bedtime.

Eating a light dinner late in the day eases your body into nighttime. Calories consumed at the close of the day simply don't burn well. Your body doesn't need much energy to sleep, and your entire metabolism begins to slow down in the late afternoon. Meals that taste good and feel filling yet don't contain a lot of calories make ideal suppers. It's also much easier to face preparing a simple meal at the end of the day than a conventional three or five course meal! For example, the Irresistible Lasagne Roll-Ups (page 95), Seaside Shell Salad (page 86), Tempting Tempeh with Soba Noodles (page 87), or any of our salads take just a few minutes to prepare, but they supply the crunch and flavor most of us crave after a hard day at work or running around after kids. These dishes also give you energy to prepare food for tomorrow's hearty lunch as you straighten up the kitchen.

Snacks need to be light, also. Sometimes our bodies and appetites tell us that an extra nosh is in order, so it's perfectly okay to snack on "upper" foods such as fruits, vegetables, grain products, or any food that is nutritious and low in fat, sugar and sodium. Carry snacks in your purse or briefcase so that you won't succumb to the temptations of vending machines or fast-food outlets. A packed snack can also come to the rescue of your energy levels when circumstances prevent you from eating a meal on time. No doubt you're aware that your brain's consciousness that it's mealtime triggers physiological responses that must be answered with food. Healthy snacks help us to maintain high energy levels. Listen to your internal cues—sensations of hunger, feelings of fatigue at odd times of the day, and dizziness—and eat when you're truly hungry. Those internal cues, signals of your circadian rhythms, usually synchronize quite naturally with your brain's knowledge that it's time for breakfast, lunch or dinner. Eating reasonable amounts of food at regular intervals will keep your whole body working smoothly and energetically. Become conscious of and learn to ignore tempting external cues—such as the sweet smells or sight of an attractive dessert—that trigger you to eat at inappropriate times. When you do eat, chew your food slowly and thoroughly, eat only in your kitchen or dining room, and focus completely on your food so that you can enjoy the texture, color, taste, and aroma of the food. Some people also benefit by arranging their meals attractively on small plates and using small utensils that prompt them to take more bites per serving. Eating while driving, sunning, working, reading, or watching television will only sabotage your natural rhythms and condition your body to believe it needs food while you're engaged in those activities. And television advertisements provide far too many provocations to eat. As you're well aware, the media—and American society in general—encourages us to reward ourselves with food or alcohol for jobs well done. We celebrate almost every event by feasting. Of course, mild food splurges on holidays are understandable and may even be psychologically necessary, but food motivates too many of us on a daily basis, and some of us live to eat instead of the other way around. The bottom line is that overeating makes you overweight.

Gaining control of your weight involves modifying your behavior so that you see food as fuel for your body rather than as a reward or security blanket. If you need to lose some pounds and fat, then begin to substitute other appealing rewards for the food bonuses you're so fond of. Try one of the following when you feel like patting yourself on the back, or even when you need a little cheering up:

- Take a leisurely drive or bike ride.
- Call a friend or relative.
- Visit a museum, zoo, or amusement park.
- Spend a night on the town—take in a concert, play or movie.
- Go dancing.
- Listen to music and buy a new CD.
- Get a new haircut or a manicure.
- Get a massage or a facial.
- Read a book.
- Spend a quiet evening propped up in bed and reading the stacks of magazines you have been meaning to peruse.
- Take an adult education course or sign up for music, art, or sports lessons.
- Investigate and begin a new hobby.
- Go shopping for clothes, shoes, or jewelry (if you can afford them!).
- Visit the ocean or the nearest lake or river and spend an afternoon relaxing in the sunshine.
- Plan and begin a new craft project.
- Purchase some new exercise equipment.
- Find yourself a pet and learn about its care and feeding.
- Visit an elderly person who would love to see you.
- Make a gift basket of toiletries or kitchen gadgets to give to a friend.
- Plan a vacation.
- Redecorate a room in your home.
- Clean house—what seems like a chore may actually rejuvenate you.

While you're at it, you may want to begin a food diary in which you record absolutely everything you eat for at least a week. Include in your diary notations about what exactly prompted you to eat. An argument with a loved one or a boss? A spell of loneliness? Exhaustion after a long day? A salary raise? A birthday celebration? Just the process of writing down what goes into your mouth will make you think twice about food choices and amounts. Such a diary will also open your eyes as to your eating patterns and maybe even help you to perceive some of your body's circadian rhythms. Even though the Double Energy Diet frees you to eat a whole range of fruits, vegetables, grains, and legumes almost indiscriminately, you'll be better equipped to withstand onslaughts of advertisements for packaged foods as well as the aromas of candy shops if you can motivate yourself to eat only what you have planned and when you are truly hungry.

One of the tricks to maintaining this kind of control of your diet is visualization, a simple technique by which you imagine a lean new you. Visualization involves daydreaming about the body you would like to have. That's not too hard, is it? Feel free to imagine yourself as a fashion model or a prize-winning athlete if it will help you set a positive goal for yourself and keep you from tossing your eating plan out of the window. Visualize how good you will feel tomorrow if you don't give in to temptation today. If you do succumb to a forbidden goodie, don't think you've blown your whole eating plan and start eating everything in sight! Simply visualize yourself back on track, eating piles of nutritious foods instead.

One of the keys to sticking with the LML Plan and maintaining that positive image of yourself is having a kitchen stocked with wholesome foods. If you maintain a good inventory of healthful ingredients, you can cook almost anything you please at a moment's notice, and you won't have to run to the store every day, only to be tempted by packaged, high-fat foods. Keep such unhealthy foods out of your pantry and refrigerator as well. If double-fudge brownies lurk in your cupboard, we'll bet they won't remain there but a day or two. Basically, do not have junk food in the house because it's too tempting. Once you train your taste buds to eat healthy foods you will not crave unhealthy foods! Here are the foods you should keep in your kitchen:

- **Flours and cereals:** whole-wheat flour, whole-wheat pastry flour, yellow cornmeal, wheat germ, oat bran, unprocessed wheat bran flakes, amaranth flour, soy flour, rice flour, bran cereal, oat cereal, flaxseeds and flaxseed meal

- **Whole grains and related foods:** barley, bulgur (cracked wheat), millet, rolled oats, brown rice, wild rice, whole grain pastas

- **Legumes, dried and/or canned:** black beans, chickpeas (garbanzo beans), kidney beans, lentils, pinto beans, soybeans, split peas, white beans (navy or Great Northern), dry-roasted and unsalted peanuts

- **Leavenings:** aluminum-free baking powder, baking soda, cornstarch, active dry yeast

- **Dried herbs and spices:** allspice, basil, bay leaves, cayenne pepper, celery seed, chili powder, cinnamon, whole and ground cloves, coriander, cumin, curry powder, dill weed, garlic powder, ground ginger, kelp, marjoram, mint leaves, mustard powder, ground nutmeg, onion powder, oregano leaves, paprika, parsley flakes, black pepper, white pepper, poppy seeds, rosemary, savory leaves, shelled sesame seeds, tarragon, thyme leaves, commercial herb blends

- **Liquid seasonings:** almond extract, vanilla extract, reduced-sodium soy sauce, Tabasco sauce, tamari, tomato paste (with no added salt), tomato sauce (choose salt-free or low-sodium sauce), vinegars, Worcestershire sauce, and Bragg Liquid Aminos (this is a healthy alternative to tamari and soy sauce)

- **Sweeteners:** apple juice concentrate, pineapple juice concentrate, applesauce, honey, molasses (preferably blackstrap), raisins, maple syrup, rice syrup, dates, pear juice concentrate and agave nectar

- **Oils:** Cold-pressed extra-virgin olive, safflower, sunflower, macadamia, peanut, canola and corn

- **Other necessary fats:** soft margarine or natural soft "buttery" spreads such as Earth Balance, which is nonhydrogenated and lactose- and gluten-free. If you keep butter in your diet, make sure it is organic. Nut butters, such as almond, peanut and cashew butter, are delicious. Read the labels on nut butters to make sure there are no hidden sweeteners, additives, or salt.

- **Fresh vegetables:** bean sprouts, broccoli and/or cauliflower, cabbage, carrots, celery, garlic, asparagus, all lettuces, spinach, mushrooms, onions, potatoes, tomatoes, plus whatever is in season

- **Fresh fruits:** apples, bananas, grapes, watermelon (all melons), peaches, plums, nectarines, papaya, pineapple, kiwi, oranges, plus whatever is in season

- **Condiments:** ketchup, mustard and mayonnaise (choose an egg-free mayonnaise such as Vegenaise)

- **Other kitchen staples:** rice or soy milk, all nuts, popcorn and whole grain crackers

The recipes in *The Double Energy Diet* are a cinch! Many of them can be prepared ahead of time, saving you last-minute work. If you get in the habit of planning your menu a few days at a time, you can streamline your shopping and food preparation further. We've included a sample seven-day menu to show you what a week's worth of healthy eating looks like. But how do you handle meals away from home?

Because friends and menus may weaken your resolve to follow the LML Plan, you will especially need your powers of visualization when you dine out. Here are a few tips for coping with restaurant food:

- Find out which restaurant you are going to ahead of time and have the restaurant fax or email you their menu, so you can decide on a healthy option in advance. Many restaurants have web sites that include their menus. If you don't have access to the menu beforehand, and you find yourself at a restaurant reading the menu, we suggest you find a dish that appeals to you, and then ask the waiter if the meal can be altered. Most restaurants are very accommodating. We have never had a problem "modifying" the dish offered. If you want to exchange the anchovy-based

Caesar salad dressing with a vinaigrette or substitute pine nuts for cheese, then just ask. Restaurants want to satisfy their patrons.

- You may wish to eat a snack before you go to a new restaurant so you won't feel ravenous and eat impulsively.

- Order mineral water, tea, spring water, or fruit juice when companions order alcoholic beverages. (See chapter 2 for our discussion of the dangers of alcohol.)

- Choose appetizers such as soups or salads that contain fresh fruits and vegetables, and request oil and vinegar or lemon and balsamic vinegar to use as alternatives for salad dressings. Beware of salad bars with creamy salad dressings. These dressings can be high in calories, sugar, and saturated fats.

- Stick to the greens and fresh fruits offered at salad bars; avoid premade salads such as slaws, pasta salads, and bean salads that may contain excessive amounts of oil, salt, hidden sugars, and preservatives. Thoroughly look over the fruits and vegetables at the salad bar. The lettuce should look crisp and green, not limp or reddish at the edges. Avoid shredded cheeses, because these contribute unnecessary fat.

- Choose light pasta dishes with tomato-based sauces instead of cream sauces.

- Ask the waiter to hold the sauce on prepared meals. Instead of rich, creamy sauces ask the waiter for shredded Parmesan cheese or some toasted nuts to place on top of the meal.

- Check the side orders on the menu. Often there are wonderful choices such as corn bread, brown rice, baked potatoes, and guacamole.

- Order vegetables raw, steamed, or stir-fried rather than deep-fried.

- If you want something sweet for dessert, order fresh fruit. Or skip dessert at the restaurant and eat a dessert at home that contains less sugar and fat.

- Ask for a "doggie bag" to take home portions of your meal that you can't finish.

Because restaurants all over the country are beginning to pay attention to the needs of health conscious diners, many now offer "heart healthy" dishes, low-fat and even low carbohydrate dishes. Chefs at reputable eating establishments are certainly accustomed to requests from diners with special dietary needs. You're paying for the meal, so don't be afraid to ask for what you want.

It's OK to splurge and try something new at a restaurant. We believe in the 90/10 rule: Eat healthfully 90 percent of the time and allow yourself some slack about 10 percent of the time. Occasionally we all stray from a healthy diet. Don't beat yourself up. But do think about how you feel after you have a huge celebration meal such as a Thanksgiving feast. If you feel tired and bloated, then you are experiencing a "food hangover." This is not fun. Just take note of how you feel after you eat foods known as "downer" foods, which have excessive amounts of sugar, fats, and additives in them. That "icky" feeling you get after eating "downer" foods will prevent you from truly ever wanting to eat them again. Just remember, if you want to have more energy and feel good, then you have to make "upper" food choices as discussed in the previous chapter.

We suggest you bring along natural digestive aid pills or ginger capsules. Country Life Vitamins puts out a vegetarian enzyme complex, called Maxi-zyme Caps, that supports maximum digestion. We take one tablet before a restaurant meal. Acti-zyme is one of many formula supplements that allows for the efficient digestion of food and maintenance of a healthy intestinal environment, and maximum absorption of nutrients. We highly recommend taking acidophilus and probiotic complex supplements, which enhance digestion and add beneficial bacteria to the body. These supplements provide naturally occurring live enzymes, vitamins, and minerals designed to optimize digestion and immunity. Primal Defense by Garden of Life is another great probiotic combination containing fourteen strains of plant-based, nondairy microorganisms that help eliminate yeast, parasites and bad bacteria from the intestines. We take probiotic supplements daily and find that they help our digestion.

The longer you follow the basic guidelines of the Double Energy Diet, the easier it will be for you to turn down unhealthy foods. Your retrained taste buds and your educated mind won't crave the foods that swell your body dimensions.

Power Through Pregnancy

PRIME TIME TO GAIN MORE ENERGY

4

Both of us agree that we didn't like being pregnant. (Although we hated the process, we loved the product.) We were often baffled when someone would say they loved being pregnant and that they never felt better. We finally figured out that many of the people who actually loved being pregnant were the people who did not take care of themselves before they became pregnant. Once they stopped smoking, drinking and/or started watching what they ate, they soon felt better.

Our children are the greatest joys in our lives and we know that the greatest gift we can give them is good health. Mothers have a responsibility to eat healthy and to feed their children healthfully. Eating healthfully during pregnancy prepares you for labor and gives your baby a healthy start in life.

The Double Energy Diet is a perfect diet for the mother-to-be. Here are some helpful guidelines to maintain optimum health and energy through pregnancy.

Don't count calories. Pregnancy is not the time to worry about the extra weight you will gain. The recommended weight gain for an average size woman is 25 to 35 pounds. When we were pregnant we gained most of our weight in the first six months. Some women gain most of their weight in their last trimester (the last three months). If you are eating healthfully, then you will gain the appropriate weight for you and your baby's health. Avoiding foods high in salt does reduce extra water retention.

Take a good prenatal vitamin. Along with a good diet, it is important to take a good prenatal vitamin. (We preferred the vitamins from the natural foods store rather than the ones the doctor prescribed because we did not like the artificial ingredients, sweeteners and binders that are commonly found in prescribed medications.) While you are pregnant, your body needs more calcium, iron, folic acid, vitamins A, C, and D, and zinc. Calcium is critical in building your baby's bones and teeth. If you don't consume enough calcium during pregnancy, the fetus will rob your calcium, putting you at risk for bone loss. A minimum of 1,200 milligrams is necessary. Dark green leafy vegetables, cottage cheese, yogurt, and skim milk are all good sources of calcium.

Iron is required to make hemoglobin, the red blood cell component that carries oxygen through the bloodstream. During pregnancy the fetus uses iron to build its own supply and more hemoglobin is required. Pregnant women need twice as much iron (about 30 milligrams a day). You can get iron from dried fruits, dried beans and pasta, whole-grain bread, and dark green leafy vegetables. Choose natural supplements, which are free of artificial flavors and colors, yeast, and preservatives. Look for non-constipating iron supplements and check with your healthcare provider about the right dose for you. Folic acid is a B vitamin that is used to produce the extra blood you and your baby need and helps in proper body enzyme function. Taken before conception and early in pregnancy, folic acid also helps prevent neural tube defects (which occur when the brain, spinal cord, or their coverings do not form normally) and cleft lip or palate (a gap in the lip or roof of the mouth). Good sources of folic acid include green leafy vegetables, broccoli, asparagus, oranges, lentils, and peanuts.

Vitamin A is necessary for healthy skin, bones and eyes and helps to create the cells that will make up your baby's internal organs. You can get all you need each day (about 2,500 IU) with just four servings of cantaloupe, carrots, dark yellow vegetables, one peach or nectarine, or a six-ounce glass of vegetable juice. Excessive levels of vitamin A (over 10,000 IU) can be harmful to you and your baby, so don't overdo it with supplements.

Vitamin C is the nutrient that helps in the manufacture of collagen, a protein that provides structure to your baby's bones, cartilage, muscles, and blood vessels. It is an antioxidant that helps prevent disease. Your body can't store Vitamin C, so it is crucial that you get the minimum amount of 65 milligrams a day. Once again, most fruits and vegetables from grapefruits to cabbage contain lots of Vitamin C.

Vitamin D helps build bone, tissue, and teeth. It enables your body to use calcium and phosphorus. You need at least 10 milligrams a day and you can get it easily from skim milk, eggs, and plenty of sunshine. (Just don't forget your sunscreen!) Zinc is the latest "must have" mineral during pregnancy. It aids fetal growth. The recommended daily dose is 20 milligrams; good sources include whole grains and dairy products.

Deal with tummy trouble. During the first trimester (the first three months), many women get nausea, also known as morning sickness. We felt nausea during our pregnancies. Morning sickness does not necessarily occur in the morning. The key to dealing with morning sickness is to eat every couple of hours. You don't need to eat a lot, but eat something. We know that is hard to do when you just want to vomit! Also, ginger helps to relieve nausea. You can get ginger tea (herbal, decaffeinated tea) at your local natural foods store and most supermarkets. If you feel queasy when you are taking your prenatal vitamin, then try taking it with your meals. Never take vitamins on an empty stomach.

Give yourself some spa time. Whether you are pregnant or not, reducing your stress level and creating some quiet time for yourself each day to recharge your battery will help you maintain your energy. We refer to this time as "spa time." It is good to take a 30-minute nap each day. Whether you are pregnant or not, good sleep habits can give you more energy. At the end of your nap, try placing cucumber slices over your closed eyelids. The cucumbers soothe your eyes and reduce under-eye puffiness. Propping pillows around your body and between your legs can help you sleep more comfortably as your belly continues to grow.

Before you take a shower at night or in the morning, give yourself a dry brush massage. A dry brush with natural bristles can be used to brush your legs and body to stimulate circulation. Begin at your feet and brush upward in long strokes on your legs towards your heart. Continue to brush on your arms and then in circular movements on your abdomen. The entire massage should take from one to five minutes. Regular brushing of the skin not only opens pores and increases cell renewal, but it also helps prevent premature aging.

Getting a massage once a month is wonderful for you during your pregnancy. Many people think of massages as a luxury, but we believe they are a necessity. Massages will help you feel relaxed, increase circulation, and soothe your muscles as your body changes.

Avoid coffee and caffeine. Drinking coffee or decaffeinated coffee during pregnancy can make you nauseous. Coffee is a diuretic, as well as a stimulant, and staying hydrated is especially important during pregnancy. Dehydration is the number one cause of fatigue in pregnant women. (Try to remember to drink at least eight glasses of water a day.) Because coffee has a dehydrating effect, it's a wise idea to avoid drinking coffee not only during pregnancy, but also if you are breastfeeding.

According to a study published in 2000 by Lisa B. Signorello, an epidemiologist at the International Epidemiology Institute in Rockville, MD, the risk of miscarriage increased twofold among pregnant Swedish women who ingested 500 milligrams or more of caffeine a day (equivalent to five cups of coffee). And some studies have shown that there is a risk to women at the 300 milligrams per day mark. Caffeine can cause many problems for pregnant women. Caffeine is not just in coffee, it is also found in chocolate and soft drinks, which we refer to "downer foods."

Stay away from trans fats. Trans fats (aka trans fatty acid) are found in hydrogenated oil. Trans fats have been linked to serious health problems including type 1 diabetes and breast cancer. They also raise the risk of heart disease by increasing LDL (bad) cholesterol and lowering HDL (good) cholesterol. According to Bridget Swinney, author of *Eating Expectantly* (Meadowbrook Press 2006) and *Healthy Food for Healthy Kids* (Meadowbrook Press 1999), trans fats pose a unique health risk for expectant and nursing moms. Studies show that women who eat high amounts of trans fats had a higher risk of experiencing preeclampsia, a dangerous complication in which blood pressure suddenly spikes. It also interferes with the body's use of omega-3 fats, which are the essential building blocks for the brain and eyes. A diet high in trans fats during pregnancy or breastfeeding can affect the development of your baby's brain and eyes. Please avoid any hydrogenated or partially hydrogenated oils. They are often found in peanut butter, hot cocoa mix, chocolate bars, microwave popcorn, flour tortillas, crackers, cookies, muffins, cereals, nut mixes, and chips. The good news is that many of these products are also made without trans fats; remember to read those labels!

Avoid certain raw foods and alcohol. Even though the Double Energy Diet does not include the consumption of any meat, fish or alcohol, we want to emphasize that pregnant women should avoid raw fish because it contains harmful bacteria. Unfortunately, our waters are polluted and many fish contain high levels of mercury, PCBs (polychlorinated biphenyls—industrial chemicals banned decades ago that are still lingering in the environment and have been linked to cancer), and other toxins. Cooking can reduce PCB levels by 30 percent (mercury cannot be reduced by cooking). Yes, fish contains omega-3 fatty acids that not only help protect against heart attacks, strokes and even rheumatoid arthritis, but are important for the baby's developing brain. However, we recommend taking omega-3 capsules or including flaxseed oil in your diet instead. The capsules and flaxseed oil contain no mercury and are toxin-free.

We suggest you avoid soft or mold-ripened cheese such as Brie or Stilton because of the risk of listeria, and avoid eating raw eggs because they may contain salmonella. Alcohol should be avoided because it could lead to fetal alcohol syndrome (FAS). FAS can cause physical and mental disabilities in a child. Children with FAS often have abnormal facial features, stunted growth, and problems with their central nervous system. In addition, they may have difficulty learning, concentrating, and communicating.

Beware of pesticides. We emphasize the importance of eating lots of fruits and vegetables. Eating certified organic produce is especially important when you are pregnant. Organic food usually costs more, but it is worth it! Paying a little extra for food can save you a ton of money on doctors' bills later. If you cannot buy organic produce, then make sure you clean your produce well with lemon juice, apple cider vinegar, sea salt water or organic produce cleaner.

Throw the death stick away. The Double Energy Diet does not allow for smoking. No woman, pregnant or not, should smoke. In fact, there should be a law banning pregnant women from smoking. Miscarriage, placental abruption, premature rupture of the membranes, premature birth, and low birth weight have all been shown to be more prevalent in pregnancies of smokers. Smoking causes vascular disease, which affects the blood flow through the placenta. Often, the placentas of smokers look older than they should because the blood vessels are calcified and partially obstructed. Placental abruption is when the placenta separates from the wall of the uterus while the fetus still needs the nutrients and oxygen. Abruption can lead to vaginal bleeding in late pregnancy, premature birth, fetal distress and even fetal death. There are so many studies that show the dangers of smoking while pregnant that no person with a conscience can legitimize smoking during her pregnancy. Please remember, secondhand smoke must be avoided, too.

Exercise for the two of you. To keep your energy up during pregnancy you must move. We found that exercising first thing in the morning kept us from feeling nausea. Getting the fresh air in your system pumps you up for the rest of the day. If you have always exercised, then you should have no problem exercising through your pregnancy. We advise women to talk to their doctor about an exercise regime. Be careful not to get your heart rate up too high or let your body get overheated. Listen to your body and do what feels comfortable. Swimming and walking don't put too much stress on your joints and are excellent exercises to do while pregnant. Many fitness clubs have special classes for pregnant women that are specifically designed for the growing waist. Exercise is not only important for you, it also gets more oxygen to your baby. Remember, your baby's health starts in the womb.

Raising Healthy Kids

GETTING OFF TO A GOOD START

In today's quick-fix, fast-paced world it may seem difficult to make sure children eat well and exercise regularly. However, it can be done, and it can be done effortlessly. Healthy eating habits are one of the most important lessons a child learns. Children basically eat what they like, and they innately know when they are full. There is never a need to push food on them. Still, it is important for parents to provide good food choices for their children.

There are several ways to encourage healthy eating habits in children. The ideal time to start kids eating healthfully is when they are infants. We can't emphasize enough the importance of breastfeeding. When our children were born we knew we were going to breastfeed them because it was the "healthy thing to do," although it was not always easy. Breastfeeding is a true art! You're probably well aware that breast milk is best for babies. However, did you know that the benefits of breastfeeding extend well beyond basic nutrition? In addition to containing all the vitamins and nutrients a baby needs in the first six months of life, breast milk is packed with disease-fighting substances that protect a baby from illness. That is why the American Academy of Pediatrics recommends exclusive breastfeeding for the first six months. Breastfeeding protects babies from gastrointestinal trouble, respiratory problems, and ear infections. Breastfeeding may even boost a child's intelligence. Several studies have found that breastfed babies are less likely to develop food or respiratory allergies. Scientists think that the fatty acids and immune factors such as IgA found in breast milk prevent allergic reactions by stopping large foreign proteins from getting into the baby's system. For some, breastfeeding is not an option, and in that case we recommend using healthy organic formulas.

As soon as babies start eating solid foods, feed them fresh fruit, vegetables and whole grains. Use a baby food grinder to grind up these foods. You can also buy ready-made baby foods at natural foods stores and supermarkets. Earth's Best is an excellent organic brand, and Gerber now puts out an organic line of baby foods. Try to get organic foods for your child, and always read the label. Children do not need extra additives, preservatives, hydrogenated oils, salts, or sugars.

Don't worry if you have an older child who didn't start out eating healthfully—it's never too late! Here are some ways to get your child eating healthy:

■ **Find out what your child likes to eat:** If the foods your child likes best are not nutritious, find healthier substitutes at your local natural foods store. There are wonderful alternatives to traditional pizzas, enchiladas, hot dogs, cheese (try soy, rice, or almond cheese), cookies, crackers (get whole grain crackers without hydrogenated oils), and other traditional snacks. Just about every unhealthy food in this universe has a healthy food alternative!

■ **Find fun recipes:** Go to your local bookstore or go online and look for healthy recipes that your child may like. Make choosing and preparing the recipe a fun family day; go the grocery store with your child, let her help select the ingredients in the recipes, and then make the food together. Most kids find cooking fun and they love to eat what they make. Helping you cook may also make your child appreciate the effort you put into buying and preparing meals.

■ **Share your concerns about eating healthy with your pediatrician, school teachers, or a close relative:** Often when a child is encouraged to eat healthfully by a respected adult other than his parent, he may "get it" better. For example, when Judi wanted her son to eat more protein, she asked her family doctor to bring up the importance of protein and discuss the foods that may be good choices for her child. Her doctor discussed the importance of eating a balanced diet including protein and encouraged her son to name protein-rich foods. Because Judi's son admired his doctor, he made an effort to eat more protein.

■ **Start an organic garden with your child:** If you don't have room for a garden, then try buying a sprout jar and seeds at your local natural foods store and grow your own sprouts at home.

■ **Go to the source:** Take your child to the local farmer's market and let him help you pick out foods and try samples.

■ **Start a reward system:** If your child tries a new food, offer a small reward like a sticker, book, or even money. However, don't bargain with food and offer desserts or sweets as a reward.

■ **Keep open communication with your child:** Older children may feel peer pressure to eat what other kids are eating so they fit in. Remember to stress the importance of good nutrition and why it's essential to eat healthy. Let kids know about the health problems, such as cancer, diabetes, heart disease, and obesity that result from not eating healthfully. Reassure your child that those who are confident about making proper food choices are actually the kids that other children admire the most. Take your younger child to a farm or zoo to see how animals that eat lots of vegetables and fruits grow big and strong.

■ **Involve your children in menu planning:** Sit down with your child to discuss what you will be putting in her school lunches and make a menu for dinners at night. For example, Monday night can be pasta night, Tuesday night can be taco night, Wednesday night can be veggie burger night, Thursday night can be pizza night, Friday night can be veggie hot dog night, and weekend dinners can be for trying new recipes.

■ **Give your child a healthy breakfast:** Breakfast is necessary to provide the nourishment and energy for an active day. Children do better in school when they start their day with a healthy breakfast. Cereals, whole-grain pancakes and waffles, and yogurt with fresh fruit are good examples of a healthy breakfast. But any healthy food can be eaten at breakfast—if your child loves salad with croutons or soup, there's nothing wrong with serving those foods for breakfast.

■ **Provide nutritious snacks:** Snacks are an important part of a child's diet because they provide necessary calories and maintain energy for children between meals. Snacks like puffed cereal, veggie sticks, fruit, cheeses, yogurts, nuts, popcorn and crackers are great food choices. Children are hungriest in the afternoon and in the evening. Children will eat what is in the house, and you can provide those smart food choices!

■ **Teach your child about "upper" and "downer" foods:** Be aware of how your child feels after he eats foods that are healthy and foods that are lacking in nutritious ingredients. When your child feels sick after eating too much candy, remind him of that "icky" feeling, and how he may not want to experience that feeling again. When your child feels energized after eating a salad or whole grain sandwich, discuss how he feels right then and there. Your child will be encouraged to pick foods that make him feel good. In chapter 2 we discuss the "upper" and "downer" foods and why in general it's better to stick with "upper" foods.

■ **Never sacrifice flavor:** All of us want to eat foods that taste good. Healthy foods are truly good tasting foods. Still, occasionally there are "throw out days" such as birthdays, holidays and other special occasions when children splurge on food. Children shouldn't be deprived of ice cream (try soy or rice-based ice creams), cake, and candy, but should rather be encouraged to eat healthier alternatives. Once a child eats healthier foods, she will on her own decline to eat "junk food."

- **Travel healthfully:** Travel with healthy foods such as nuts, crackers and popcorn. Having those healthy foods available will help you make better food choices on a road trip. Also, if you are at a restaurant, you may want to skip the "kids' menu" items. Often, kids' menus consist of French fries and pasta drenched in butter and are higher in fat than the regular menu. Bring bottled water with you when you travel on airplanes. Use it not only for drinking, but also for brushing teeth and washing face and hands. Airplane water is not worth drinking.

- **Consider children's vitamins and supplements:** Some children could use a nutritional boost. There are wonderful children's multiple vitamins and vitamin drinks that children can choose from. For instance, Alacer corporation makes drink mix packets called Emer'gen C. These drinks have Vitamin C, mineral complexes, antioxidants and several vitamins. They are sweetened with fructose and come in fun flavors such as strawberry, tangerine, raspberry, orange and lemon lime. Just add these packets of powder to water and to get a nutritious fizzing drink mix.

- **Encourage your child to drink water:** Make sure you put a water bottle in your child's lunch and backpack. When we pick up our children from school we actually have water in a cooler ready for them in the car. Water is important for people of all ages to drink.

- **Get moving:** Since 1980, the percentage of overweight children has doubled, and the percentage of overweight adolescents has nearly tripled! Overweight children stand a higher risk of getting asthma, type 2 diabetes, heart disease, and bone and joint problems. But children love to play and move and sometimes need just a little encouragement to exercise.

Go on family bike rides and hikes, and play sports with your children. Offer to be a coach on your child's sports team. Not only will you have fun exercising together, but your child will feel so proud to have you there! The benefits of exercise are tremendous for people of all ages. Diet and exercise go hand and hand to maintain a healthy lifestyle. Vigorous physical activity is vital to good health. Get kids involved in sports that interest them.

These are a few ways to encourage children to live a healthier, more energized lifestyle. Remember, the best way to teach is by example.

Exercise 6

THE ULTIMATE ENERGY BOOSTER

When we tell you that exercise is absolutely essential to your success for maintaining optimal energy, please don't wince. You already know that exercise is supposed to be good for you, but every time you start a new exercise program, your appetite seems to skyrocket. You assume that exercise is simply inviting bigger food bills and bigger bulges, and you tell yourself that physical activity will only make you feel more fatigued than usual. So you quit running or swimming or walking—or whatever sport you tried this time around.

Convincing your sedentary self that you've made the right decision seems especially easy after you hear proponents of crash diets proclaim that exercise in itself won't burn enough calories to make a dent in your excess fat. (And taking off one pound of flesh does require a lot of effort—about sixteen hours of bicycling or fast walking!) Advocates of quickie diets assert that the only way to lose weight is to eat fewer calories.

Trouble is, crash dieters, who may indeed lose weight quickly, tend to feel exhausted because they are depriving their bodies of fuel. Furthermore, they simply pile the pounds back on when they return to their normal eating habits. Too often, perennial dieters pack on more fat than they carried before their last diets. Fat propagates fat, and dieters who are temporarily successful but who normally carry too much fat will still tend to turn most of the food they eat into fat because they haven't developed any lean muscle tissue, the substance that works to remove body fat. Unfortunately, many dieters who lose weight will eventually regain it. This is why a diet should be thought of as a lifestyle.

Low-calorie diets make our bodies fight to maintain what medical researchers now call the set point, the weight at which the human body stabilizes when its owner is not actively trying to gain or lose weight. When faced with calorie deficits, the area in our brains that regulates how much body fat we carry begins to panic, so it increases our appetites and clamps down our metabolisms so that we don't burn food calories or fat as well as we did before. Moreover, radical weight reduction diets can change body chemistries for the worse: although they will trigger weight loss, crash diets may actually raise set points and lower basal metabolic rates, the speed at which our bodies burn calories while we're at rest.

Yes, adhering to a lose-it-quick eating program lets you peel off pounds rapidly— but only at the diet's outset. The first weight to come off consists of water and muscle, body components much more easily shed than pounds of fat, each of which stores twice the number of calories as a pound of glycogen (carbohydrate storage) or protein. After the first five or ten pounds drop away, weight loss slows down, and your body struggles to conserve stored energy. It's not easy to keep the weight off on these fad diets. You may get pretty tired of limited food choices and calorie or "carb" counting, and your body weight will bounce up and down as you diet, regain, diet, regain, ad infinitum.

But here's the flip side of the story: researchers have found in repeated studies that exercise improves body chemistry. Indeed, exercise will lower your body's set point and raise your basal metabolic rate. Even if you eat the same amount as you did before you began to exercise, you'll lose weight. No joke! Dr. Dennis Remington, an obesity expert at Brigham Young University, theorizes that the body somehow senses that an active person needs to be thin and lowers the body's set point.

Now that you understand how physical exertion can transform your metabolism, give exercise an honest try. You'll notice that your appetite may decrease for a couple of hours after you exert yourself, and then increase an hour or two later. However, your body's lowered set point will give you a feeling of greater control over your appetite, and you'll burn off food calories more quickly than you did before. There's a bonus, too: not only do you burn calories and body fat during strenuous exercise, but you continue to burn more calories than usual for hours after exercise because vigorous activity boosts your basal metabolic rate, making it hard for your body to conserve energy in the form of fat. In fact, a team of scientists recently found that intense exercise stimulated calorie expenditure up to nine hours later, and lipid oxidation, or the burning of fat, for at least eighteen hours after the subjects had stopped exercising.

And body fat is the issue here; losing anything other than body fat can be harmful. As Covert Bailey points out in his scientifically grounded, enormously popular book *Fit or Fat?* (Houghton Mifflin 1978), being overweight only signals that you are carrying too much fat, and people who think they're maintaining an ideal weight may be fat, too. The older you are, the more likely it is that your muscles have begun to turn to fat. The scales tell only a partial truth; the tape measure tells you a bit more. For example, two people who weigh the same may be incredibly different in terms of fitness. One may be trim and muscular, and the other may exhibit rolls around the middle or pouches on the thighs. Part of the reason for this discrepancy in appearance is that the lean muscle on the first person weighs more than the fat that pads the second. In addition, all bodies carry muscle in a neater fashion than they do fat.

Interestingly, researchers have proven that most heavy people don't eat more than thin people do; people who carry too much fat simply move less and have lower basal metabolic rates. Instead of using food fuel in vigorous movement, their bodies, which possess relatively little lean muscle, convert food fuel to fat. The only way that overly fat people can succeed at weight loss programs and then sustain a nearly ideal weight is to lower their set points and raise their metabolic rates permanently by involving themselves in a regular exercise program. How do you know if you're too fat? Don't rely on the scale. Take a look in the mirror; check to see if you've got extra padding where you don't want it. How do your clothes fit? Can you pinch several inches of skin on the back of your upper arm? As we previously mentioned, every body needs fat to cushion organs, to metabolize certain vitamins, and to store energy for emergency purposes; however, more than a little fat is not good.

Drastically reducing your calorie intake will cause your body to burn unnecessary fat eventually, but such deprivation saps energy and works against muscle gain. In contrast, exercising regularly will pump up adrenaline levels and help you lose fat gradually and effectively. As we explained above, exercise creates the lean muscle that metabolizes fat all over your body. In case you didn't know it, there's no such thing as so-called spot reducing. You can tone up the muscles in a specific area, but the only way to lose fat in a certain spot is to exercise energetically. Of course, there are people who resort to the "short cuts" in life and get plastic surgery to remove fat, but we don't think this is healthy for the body.

There are two main types of exercise, aerobic and anaerobic, but only aerobic exercise burns fat and helps you lose weight. Aerobic exercise involves continuous movement of large muscle groups that send signals to the heart and lungs to circulate lots of oxygen. ("Aero" is the Greek word for air.) Because your muscles need oxygen to burn fat (and carbohydrates) it's important to have plenty of oxygen circulating through your body. Activities that can be aerobic include the following: brisk walking, hiking, jogging, running, dancing, rowing, jumping rope, cross country skiing, swimming, cycling, skating, soccer, basketball, racquetball, and handball.

To get rid of excess body fat, you must perform aerobic exercise for at least thirty-five minutes at least four times a week. You should be moving continuously and your heart should be beating at its ideal training rate, which is between 70 and 85 percent of its maximum rate, for at least twenty minutes. Sound too complicated? Actually, it's pretty simple to tell when you're exercising aerobically. First, determine your maximum heart rate (MHR), the fastest your heart should ever beat:

220 − Age = Maximum heart rate (MHR) per minute

Next, multiply your MHR by both 70 percent and 85 percent:

$$\text{MHR} \times .70 = \text{Minimum training heart rate (THR) per minute}$$

$$\text{MHR} \times .85 = \text{Maximum training heart rate (THR) per minute}$$

If your heart rate falls below the lower figure, your muscles are not burning fat. If your heart rate exceeds the higher figure, you are exercising too hard and putting too great a strain on your heart. Paradoxically, exercising too intensely may cause muscle loss. To determine your heart rate at any time, put a couple of fingers in the groove next to your Adam's apple, or place your middle finger on your wrist at your pulse point. Count the beats for six seconds, and multiply by ten. If you do this while you're exercising, keep your legs moving to keep your heart rate elevated.)

You can also tell whether you're exercising too hard by seeing if you can talk while you're in the middle of your chosen sport. If you've worked up a reasonable sweat and are breathing hard, but you can still talk to a companion, you're probably safely within your heart's training zone. We are fortunate to live in the same town so every day we try to run together. We run and talk the whole way. We call this "exercise therapy." Having an exercise buddy can make the activity even more enjoyable.

Aerobic exercise has added benefits, especially for women: such sports help prevent osteoporosis by building muscles and increasing bone density. And when women couple weight-bearing exercise with menus from *The Double Energy Diet* they significantly reduce their chances of developing osteoporosis because lacto-ovo vegetarian diets also prevent bone mineral loss.

Anaerobic exercise is important, too. Anaerobic (meaning "without air") exercises involve short spurts of energy that don't sufficiently work the lungs and heart to burn fat. Anaerobic exercise such as weight lifting, tennis, bowling, and sprinting can improve flexibility, coordination, and balance, and strengthen your muscles.

Everyone makes time to eat, so changing your diet doesn't seem to tax your schedule the way altering your fitness level does. How can you find any time at all to exercise? You begin an exercise program slowly, and you gradually increase the frequency and duration of your workout times. You choose activities that appeal to you, and vary your exercise menu so that you don't get bored.

Listen to your circadian rhythms (discussed in chapter 3) to find the time of day that will work best for you. We highly recommend exercising first thing in the morning. We have been running every morning for over 20 years, and we believe that by exercising first thing in the morning we not only feel better, but we have significantly more energy throughout the day. (Yes, putting out energy gives you more energy!) The air is fresher in the morning, too. Working out first thing in the morning jump-starts us for the rest of the day, and we feel so good about ourselves knowing we have the discipline to do it. We laugh at how we feel about exercising, as we can't wait to do it, and we can't wait till it's done.

However, some people just aren't "morning" people, and if you don't like to exercise in the morning, then do it when it works for you. It's worse to not exercise at all! If you're aiming to lose fat rather than just to maintain your current fitness level, then exercise before breakfast or at least two hours after your last meal: that way, your muscles will burn fat rather than the food you just ate. Or take a deserved exercise break right after lunch when you're feeling drowsy; get your adrenaline pumping to rev up your system and activate your mind.

No matter which exercise you choose or what time of day you intend to do it, just be faithful to your plan. Remember to exercise aerobically at least four times a week for at least thirty-five minutes at a time. Those thirty-five minutes will allow you to warm up for about ten minutes, maintain your training heart rate for twenty minutes, and then cool down for another five or ten minutes. In addition to those thirty-five minutes, take a few minutes to perform some relaxed, non-bouncing stretches both before and after your regular workout. Stretching promotes flexibility and allows your muscles to ease into and out of demanding activities, preventing injury. You may also wish to supplement aerobic exercise with muscle-building anaerobic exercise. Every other day add some strength training to your workout. We do about ten minutes of light weights. Five- to ten-pound dumbbells work well. We do a bench press, overhead press, bent over press and a tricep curl with three sets of ten repetitions on each arm.

If you have trouble motivating yourself to exercise, find a "body buddy" and make a pact to exercise together consistently. Join a fitness club or a community or office team; an upbeat environment and enthusiastic teammates will excite you about your sport. Or try buying and purchasing some stylish workout outfits and shoes, and enjoy wearing them whenever you exercise.

After a few weeks on an aerobic exercise program, most people find that exercise becomes addictive, and they feel depressed or tired when they don't exercise. This beneficial addiction probably occurs because physical activity stimulates the production of beta-endorphin, a natural tranquilizer and pain-reducer that mimics the effects of morphine, the strong pain-killing narcotic. Because regular aerobic exercise gives you a natural "high," you are less likely to suffer from depression, anxiety, anger, and other everyday negative emotions. Furthermore, regular aerobic exercise dramatically improves the circulatory and elimination systems, and it decreases LDL ("bad") and increases HDL ("good") cholesterol (a process we explained in chapter 2). It also helps battle diabetes by lowering blood sugar levels, fights arthritis by enhancing the condition of joints, and improves sleep and increases daytime efficiency because it decreases anxieties and tensions.

Medical researchers continue to discover the ways in which aerobic exercise benefits our bodies and our minds. When you combine consistent aerobic exercise with complex-carbohydrate menus like those in this book, you will no doubt elevate your physical energy and enhance your mental efficiency in ways that scientists have not even documented yet.

Maintaining Double Energy

SUCCESSFUL STRATEGIES FOR CONTINUED STAMINA SUCCESS

7

ecoming a healthier person by eating well and exercising consistently may seem an agonizing procedure to those of you with potentially harmful habits. However, a willingness to take small, calculated steps rather than big, impulsive leaps toward the goal of double energy can make the process easy and pleasant. In fact, you'll become quite proud of the personal transformation you have gone through, and your gradually increasing energy will amply reward your efforts.

Nonetheless, we'll admit that acquiring and maintaining a large measure of physical energy takes more than simply eating nutritious complex carbohydrates and exercising aerobically and regularly. Sustaining an energetic, exciting lifestyle also requires a positive view of life and of yourself, a willingness to change and to accept responsibility for your own health, an appreciation of other people, and an awareness of environmental hazards and benefits.

A positive view of life and of yourself

You've heard plenty of clichés about positive mental attitudes, and you may simply ignore advice on this subject because it seems trite. Yet you can't succeed at any diet or plan for better living if you're the type of person who looks at any goal skeptically or who focuses on your failures rather than on what you've accomplished and what you can still achieve. And if you can't muster a sense of humor—if you can't summon a good, body-healing belly laugh now and then—your stress levels will probably become dangerous to your physical health.

You need to develop confidence in the Double Energy Diet and in yourself if you want to multiply your physical energy and prevent disease. Harboring too many suspicions about the diet or thoughts that you might not succeed will program you for failure.

Developing a positive mental attitude about whatever project you've undertaken involves appreciating yourself and your capabilities. Focusing on the qualities you lack rather than on your assets will only undermine your efforts. Forget about comparing yourself to another person or to some image of perfection. Accept who you are now, and find ways to grow and improve. Loving yourself will free your mind to focus on your life's tasks—including increasing and then maintaining your energy.

We'll bet you know at least a few people whose feelings of inadequacy inhibit them every hour of every day. Unhappy with some aspect of their appearance or personality, they convey that dissatisfaction to other people, thereby influencing others to see them in the same way they see themselves. Full of inner turmoil, people with negative self images tend to experience more than the usual number of conflicts in their personal relationships. In addition, their poor self-confidence makes them feel wearier than they might otherwise. Almost every task tires them.

In contrast, those who possess self-confidence, who work on but simultaneously de-emphasize their own faults and failures, attract friends and admiration. Because they can laugh at and accept themselves, they often feel energetic and practically unconquerable. Such individuals create their own possibilities, and they make the perfect (but certainly not the only) recruits for the Double Energy Diet.

A willingness to change and to accept responsibility for health

Those who cannot accept themselves are often the same people who fear change or who believe themselves the victims of circumstance. Such individuals make poor candidates for any kind of diet or exercise plan. Furthermore, they are the people who succumb to serious illness when it strikes.

Many medical doctors have observed just how crucial a patient's attitude and flexibility are to the healing process. You're probably familiar with human interest stories about people who have overcome critical illnesses almost by sheer force of will. Norman Cousins and his battle with a near-terminal illness is a prime example. Determined not to surrender to his disease, Cousins watched hours of Marx Brothers films and *Candid Camera* reruns, and he laughed his way to good health. He documents his miraculous journey back to health in the enormously popular book, *Anatomy of an Illness as Perceived by the Patient* (W.W. Norton & Co. 2005).

Dr. Bernie Siegel, a physician who works with terminally ill cancer patients, has likewise witnessed how an individual's willingness to change and to take responsibility for his or her health may prolong life or even save it. In his inspirational best seller titled *Love, Medicine and Miracles* (Harper & Row 1986), Siegel explains that "many people don't make full use of their life force until near-fatal illness guides them into a "change of mind." Part of this change usually involves learning to love oneself, as Dr. Siegel states so well:

> The fundamental problem most people face is an inability to love themselves, having been unloved by others during some crucial period in their lives. This period is almost always childhood, when our relations with our parents establish our characteristic ways of reacting to stress. As adults we repeat these reactions and make ourselves vulnerable to illness, and our personalities often determine the specific nature of the illnesses. The ability to love oneself, combined with the ability to love life, fully accepting that it won't last forever, enables one to improve the quality of life.

Long before illness strikes, those who feel unloved and have low self-esteem experience excessive fatigue. Negative images of themselves and feelings of helplessness make such people vulnerable to outside stresses and cause them to feel weary. Even if they are eating well and exercising regularly, their sense of hopelessness can negate their attempts to become healthy.

On the other hand, those who love themselves somehow recognize that potential for change lies inside them and that to some extent they can shape their worlds. Acceptance of self leads to interest in the world and to the realization that change is stimulating and challenging rather than frightening and dangerous. The individual who takes care of his or her body can see crises as opportunities for growth. This is a person whose energy levels will rise to meet whatever challenges he or she faces.

If you struggle with feelings of helplessness, or if you feel too comfortable with the status quo, at least begin to recognize the mental obstacles you've created for yourself. Perceiving a problem is half the struggle. When you can see negative emotions in yourself, you can address them and then release them. It's perfectly human and okay to feel bad about yourself once in a while, but experiencing chronic feelings of inadequacy can paralyze you.

Once you realize that you need to gain control of your life, take small steps toward enhanced appearance and health, increased energy and greater happiness. What kinds of steps do we mean? In the case of dietary and exercise goals, altering ingrained habits can be painlessly simple if you attempt one modification at a time. For example, try substituting brown rice for your usual white rice. When you need a snack, eat an apple or a whole-grain cookie instead of a candy bar. Walk for a half-hour during your lunch break: breathe deeply and notice your surroundings. When you've accepted a challenge once, try making that same change every other day—or every day. What was once different will become comfortably routine, and you will begin to sense the choices you can make about much larger aspects of your life.

Keeping a positive outlook will help you feel good inside and out, and we suggest you start thinking optimally, too. In *Optimal Thinking, How to Be Your Best Self* (John Wiley & Sons 2002), Rosalene Glickman describes optimal thinking as the language of your highest self. It empowers you to be your best and stops you from settling for second best. Basically you are being the best you can be every day. Optimal thinkers ask themselves, what is the best solution? Am I taking the smartest actions towards my goal? Am I maximizing my options? And what's the most constructive use of my time right now? For example, as an optimal thinker who is lacking energy you would ask yourself, what is the best way for me to have more energy? Then you would seek the best solution by doing research on the topic of energy. You might go to the library, book store, your family doctor, or on the internet to seek ways to have more energy. Optimal thinkers don't wait for things to happen, they make things happen. Congratulations, you are being an optimal thinker right now by reading this book!

An appreciation of other people

Accepting yourself and feeling in control of your own life will open your mind to love other people, and that love will energize your whole being and make you less vulnerable to illness.

Numerous studies have indicated that people who live in harmony with others experience far fewer bouts with disease and have greater longevity than those who feel in conflict with the world. Harmonious personal relationships bring us all kinds of energy. Skeptical? Just consider how far you'll travel to see a loved one, or how late you'll stay up to make something special for a favorite relative.

Now recall how your body usually feels when you're angry or resentful about another person's actions. These emotions are perfectly natural, but you can learn to release them by making the other person aware of the problem and/or by recognizing that the other person's actions were actually masked requests for your love and attention. Of course, we're simplifying tremendously here, and you need to consult a counselor if you're carrying around a load of anger and resentment. Nonetheless, we can tell you that forgiveness, even if it is unspoken, is a powerful tool for healing and for regaining your own energy.

It's easy to feel energized by happy, kind people. Don't waste your time hanging out with people who are depressed, mean or angry. Some people will zap your "good energy" if you let them. Stay clear from people who "bring you down," judge you or don't encourage you. People are inspired by other inspirational individuals. Think about it: when you spend time with people who are depressed and negative it makes you feel weak, but if you spend your time with people who make you laugh and feel good, then you have more energy. Energy is contagious!

An awareness of environmental hazards and benefits

Changing yourself and relating positively with others may seem surprisingly easy compared to dealing with physical hazards over which you have little control. But once you become aware of potential problems—contaminated food or water and polluted air, for example—you can make choices that will better your life and elevate your energy.

Learn where the produce you buy originates and how it is cultivated. Find out about your water supply and how its managers treat it chemically. Read about the level of pollutants in the air you breathe. If any of your discoveries troubles you, then consider buying your food from natural foods stores or directly from organic growers. Find out if there's a farmer's market in your town where local farmers sell their foods. If the weather permits, consider starting your own garden. If the area you live in has excessive levels of air pollutants, then maybe it's time to move. Do what you can to take charge of your health and that of your family.

Indoor and outdoor air quality are both important for maintaining better health and vitality. Choose household products, furnishings, paints and flooring that are made with natural or nontoxic materials. Household plants can also help clean the air by removing gases such as benzene, carbon dioxide, carbon monoxide, cigarette smoke, formaldehyde, and ozone. Popular indoor plants are bamboo, aloe vera, chrysanthemums, dracaena palms, English ivy, golden pothos, Janet Craig, philodendrons, scheffleras, and spider plants. Living in a nontoxic home is truly being energy efficient.

Indoor air quality can be altered by mold. Mold can produce allergens (substances that can cause allergic reactions). Inhaling or touching mold spores can cause severe allergic reactions. Check around wet, dark areas in your home or workplace that may harbor mold. Toxic mold can be very harmful and energy depleting.

If you live in a particularly smoggy area, you may want to invest in an air filter or a negative ion machine for your home. Ions are electrically charged atoms or clusters of atoms. A positive ion (cation) results when a neutral atom or atom cluster loses an electron, which is a negatively charged particle; a negative ion (anion) results when an atom or atom cluster gains an electron. Pollution reduces the number of oxygen and hydrogen atoms available in the air, and it causes an imbalance in the ratio of negative and positive ions. Dry winds, known as the Santa Anas here in California, carry an excess number of positive ions. Their presence makes people experience headaches, earaches, irritability, drowsiness, dry skin, and so forth. On the other hand, the presence of water, composed of hydrogen and oxygen atoms, indicates the existence of large numbers of negative ions, which scientists attribute with energizing properties. Have you ever gotten flashes of insight while you were showering or before a rainfall? Maybe you've noticed that a vacation near the ocean has made you feel particularly rejuvenated. Many people enjoy having decorative water fountains in their home because they claim they make them feel energized.

Your attitudes toward life, yourself, the people around you, and your environment can greatly affect your chances for achieving a lifetime of boundless energy. Here are some more strategies to help you sustain an exciting and energetic lifestyle:

■ **Maintain good posture and breathe correctly.** Good posture keeps the body's circulatory system working efficiently. Stand and sit up straight and breathe deep. Keep the energy flowing!

Breathing properly is important. The more deeply you breathe, the greater the amount of oxygen you send to your brain and the more energy you feel. The Chinese call the vital energy within each of us *chi*, and they call the art of manipulating one's breath *chi kung* (inner vigor), a discipline that reflects their belief that air fuels inner energy. You can learn what the Chinese have long known by practicing meditation, yoga, martial arts, Pilates, and/or stress management. Learning to breathe abdominally can bring all sorts of benefits, including a clear mind and more energy.

Whether you take a yoga class or a Lamaze class, the emphasis is on breathing. Proper breathing can tame your stress responses, sharpen your awareness, diminish pain and increase your energy. Stand up straight, don't shrug your shoulders, and exhale slowly. Then breathe slowly back in with your chest area expanding. This expands your diaphragm by pushing your stomach down and out. Do this several times whenever you feel stressed or tired.

■ **Fight fatigue with alternative medicine.** These days, if you're trying to get healthy or increase your energy you have a wide array of alternative therapies to choose from—chiropractic medicine, acupuncture, acupressure, aromatherapy, massage therapy, flower remedies, and homeopathy, to name a few. Because we are into preventive medicine we get chiropractic adjustments once a year to keep our bodies in line. We suggest getting referrals and doing research first on any practitioner you're considering working with. At the end of this book we've included a section called "The Twins' Click Picks," which lists some outstanding web sites to check out for helpful information about the benefits of alternative medicine.

■ **Create a "to do" list.** Every day make a "to do" list. Write down things you are planning to do during the day. You can write down a lunch date, a business appointment or even folding laundry; there is no task too trivial. We all need a purpose in life, and accomplishing "mini goals" every day makes you feel good and productive which, in turn, energizes you.

■ **Listen to music.** Research shows that music can affect brain wave patterns and can be an effective tool for healing. People often listen to music while driving on road trips to keep them going for their long drives. There is energy in a party that has music playing as opposed to a party without music. Faster paced music can really get you moving! Feel free to dance to the tunes and enjoy the enhanced energy you will receive from the music.

■ **Dress for success.** It's exciting to wear a new outfit or get dressed up for a special event. Wear clothes that you love and that are comfortable. If you feel attractive in your clothes, you will have more confidence in your appearance. Having confidence can boost your energy to higher levels.

■ **Pamper yourself.** Massages, facials, and pedicures rejuvenate the body. Massage increases circulation, bringing more oxygen to the body. It not only feels great, but it is great for obtaining more energy!

■ **Create energy in your interiors.** Shari is a Professional ASID Certified Interior Designer and she understands how one's interiors can truly affect one's disposition and energy. Having a home that you are proud of and enjoy brings you happiness and energy. If you have too much clutter in your house and your home is literally an obstacle course, then it's time to consider getting rid of all the items you aren't using anymore. When you give, you feel good and in turn you have more energy. For example, if you go into your closet and you see clothes that you don't wear anymore, then give them to a charitable organization (get a receipt from the charitable organization and get the tax write-off).

We believe strongly in the traditions of feng shui (pronounced "fung shway"). Feng shui literally means "wind-water" in Chinese and has become one of the hottest design trends around. Feng shui has been around since the fourth century BC when the Chinese invented the compass. During the following century, they began using the device to aid in the proper placement of grave and home sites. They believed that finding the best final resting place for their ancestors ensured health, harmony and prosperity for the descendants because we are all connected by cosmic, universal energy called "chi." Feng shui is based on these fundamental concepts: flow of energy, balance of yin and yang, and the interaction of five elements.

The flow of energy in any room is important. In nature, we find perfectly straight lines in only short segments such as in the canes of sugar or bamboo. Even the tallest redwoods have irregularities. It is a natural law that energy flows in wavy lines like the water in streams. So avoid sharp, straight edges in your home in order to keep the energy flowing. This goes for the outside of the house, too. For example, rather than a long, straight path from the street to the entry, it is better to have a path with a gentle curve. This creates a better energy flow and is believed to create more prosperity. Proper placement of furniture also makes a difference in the energy of the room; it should allow for easy movement. For instance, a large piece of furniture such as a sofa, placed with its back to the entrance of a room, automatically blocks the energy flow in that room.

Yin and yang represent the duality of the universe. Yin is the female side, the dark color of the symbol, and the yang is the male side, the light color of the symbol. Together yin and yang comprise a whole, and yet there is an element of each in the other. But sometimes we have too much yang and other times we have too much yin. It is up to us to find and maintain the balance between the two in our physical, mental, emotional, spiritual, sexual, and intellectual selves. Achieving this balance helps us become grounded and centered, much like a rock that is pounded by the elements and still remains unyielding.

The five elements are fire, earth, metal, water, and wood. These elements all work together to create energy in our lives, and it is best to balance these materials in your home to create a harmonious environment.

There are several books on feng shui that go into more detail about how to arrange furniture and the use of design elements like mirrors and plants to increase prosperity and energy in a home. A well-designed, clutter-free home will truly give you more energy.

■ **Check out your bed.** A good night's sleep is vital in order to have maximal energy throughout the day. According to the National Sleep Foundation, over one half of the American work force reports that sleepiness on the job interferes with the amount of work they get done, and 40 percent of adults admit that the quality of their work suffers when they're sleepy. A good mattress and mattress pad can make a difference in getting a successful night's sleep. Latex mattresses are derived from the sap of rubber trees and are made with no synthetic blends of styrene butadiene (SRB). The pure, natural rubber latex is resistant to mold, mildew, and bacteria. Plus, dust mites will not live in a natural rubber environment. Latex mattresses absorb approximately 85 percent of normal sleeping movements, to guarantee an undisturbed night's sleep. Look for a natural mattress with 100 percent organic ticking and batting. Lifekind is one company that offers this type of mattress.

Hypoallergenic memory foam mattress toppers can also be a wonderful way to get a good night's sleep. Memory foam has a gel-like feel that is temperature sensitive; the warmth of your body softens the mattress. It recognizes shape and pressure points and adjusts to distribute your body weight evenly.

■ **Carry a water spritzer.** Carry a small water sprayer or an atomizer (Evian water makes these) with you in your car or purse. When you feel tired just squirt some water on your face. It will not only give you an energy boost, but it's good for your skin, too!

■ **Avoid additives and preservatives.** The FDA allows more than 3,000 additives to be used in foods. The side effects of many additives may not appear until fifteen to thirty years after they're first ingested. We assimilate these additives into our bodies over time and, depending on how healthy one's immune system is, the effects can be deadly. Food additives can be carcinogenic, contribute to heart, lung and kidney disease, contribute to allergies, and cause birth defects. The Internal Agency for Research on Cancer (which is part of the World Health Organization) considers such additives as BHA and BHT to be carcinogenic. Red dye # 3, used to color pistachios, has been linked to thyroid cancer in lab rats. Additives can inhibit your stomach's ability to digest food, not only causing indigestion, but also wreaking havoc on your liver and kidneys, which are your body's detoxifying organs. You are what you eat, so read those labels!

■ **Let there be light.** Put on your sunscreen and visor, and go outside and enjoy the sun. Light stimulates neurotransmitters in the brain, such as serotonin and dopamine, that can improve your mood and increase your motivation. Exposure to any sunlight can provide a little boost. So let light energize your life!

■ **Practice dry brush massage.** Increase your energy by using a dry brush to massage yourself. Brushing your body using a long-handled brush with natural or vegetable bristles removes dead skin cells and increases blood circulation all over your body, thereby encouraging your lungs to up your oxygen intake and thus to elevate your energy levels. Every morning, use long strokes that begin at your feet and legs and move up to your neck, and be sure that your brush is completely dry.

As you see from our discussion in this chapter, many different factors affect your energy level and your spirits. Eating the "upper" foods and avoiding the "downer" foods described in chapter 2 of this book, following the LML Plan, and exercising aerobically and consistently can certainly double your energy and improve your health and appearance. However, to enjoy the full benefits of these life-changing practices, you need to accompany them with mental openness and a decision to grow in all facets of your life. Such a conscious choice can lead not only to a personal transformation but to a transformation of the world around you.

These recipes are not only nutritious and delicious, but fun and easy to make, too. The combination of fresh tastes, textures, and colors allows these recipes to burst with flavor.

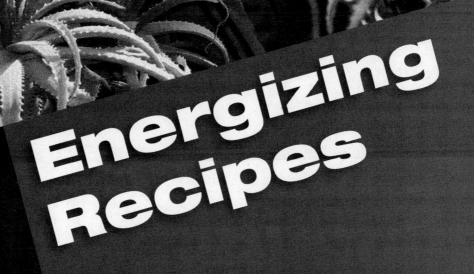

Energizing Recipes

Light Breakfasts and Healthy Treats

8

We include pies and cookies in our breakfast section because eating these sweet treats in the morning provides you with energy that you can burn off all day, which is better than eating them late at night.

BREAKFAST & TREATS

NOTE: Please check the glossary on page 135 for information about using liquid sweeteners of your choice and dairy or nondairy ingredients in recipes.

DOUBLE YOUR ENERGY **health drink**

YIELD: 1 SERVING

We have many versions of this energy drink. It is quick and filled with complex carbohydrates that are utilized by the body at a slow, steady rate.

2 large scoops dairy or nondairy ice cream

¼ cup dairy or nondairy milk

1 ripe banana

2 Oatmeal Raisin Cookies (page 61)

2 tablespoons wheat germ

2 tablespoons raw sunflower seeds

2 tablespoons nutritional yeast

2 tablespoons flaxseed meal

rocess all the ingredients in a blender for about 30 seconds. Enjoy!

VARIATIONS

Add a handful of ice cubes before blending to give the drink a frosty texture. Add ½ cup strawberries, raspberries, pineapple chunks, or blueberries—each fruit creates a distinctive flavor. Or add 2 tablespoons peanut butter for flavor and protein.

oatmeal raisin COOKIES

YIELD: 5 DOZEN COOKIES

Oatmeal and raisins complement one another in flavor and nutrition. Oatmeal has antioxidant compounds called avenanthramides, which prevent free radicals from damaging LDL cholesterol and also reduce the risk of cardiovascular disease. Raisins contain the mineral boron, which provides protection against osteoporosis.

2 tablespoons flaxseed meal

½ cup warm water

⅔ cup nonhydrogenated vegan margarine or canola oil

¾ cup liquid sweetener of your choice

1 tablespoon vanilla extract

3 cups rolled oats

1½ cups whole-wheat pastry flour

1 cup raisins

⅔ cup chopped walnuts

1 tablespoon ground cinnamon

1 teaspoon baking powder

Preheat the oven to 350 degrees F. Stir the flaxseed meal into the warm water and let sit for 5 minutes. Oil 2 baking sheets. Beat the margarine, sweetener, and vanilla together until creamy. Stir in the flaxseed mixture. Add the remaining ingredients and mix well. Drop 12 teaspoon-sized balls of dough onto each prepared baking sheet. Bake for 12 minutes, or until light golden brown. Let the cookies cool on a wire rack. Repeat with the remaining dough.

VARIATION

Add 1 cup carob chips, unsweetened shredded coconut, or pecans for a delicious twist.

ALMOND **cookies**

YIELD: 2 DOZEN COOKIES

These almond cookies are a wonderful snack in the afternoon accompanied by decaffeinated green tea. You can chop the almonds in a food processor or a blender.

1 tablespoon flaxseed meal

¼ cup warm water

⅓ cup nonhydrogenated vegan margarine

⅓ cup liquid sweetener of your choice, plus extra for dipping

2 teaspoons almond extract

1 cup whole-wheat pastry flour

½ cup coarsely chopped dry roasted almonds

12 whole almonds, split in half

Preheat the oven to 350 degrees F. Stir the flaxseed meal into the warm water and let sit for 5 minutes. Oil 2 baking sheets. Mix the margarine, sweetener, flaxseed mixture, and almond extract together. Add the flour and chopped almonds and stir to blend. Drop 12 teaspoon-sized spoonfuls of dough onto each prepared baking sheet. If desired, dip the almond halves in sweetener. Place one almond half on the center of each cookie. Bake 10 minutes, or until light golden brown. Let the cookies cool on a wire rack.

yummy apple FLAX MUFFINS

These muffins are so moist and good (and they're good for you, too). Apples are one of the eight great energy foods we discuss in chapter 2.

½ cup warm water

¾ cup plus 2 tablespoons flaxseed meal

3 green apples (Pippin or Granny Smith), peeled and shredded

¾ cup dairy or nondairy milk

½ cup liquid sweetener of your choice

1 tablespoon vanilla extract

1½ cups unbleached pastry flour

¾ cup oat bran

1 tablespoon ground cinnamon

1 teaspoon baking powder

½ cup raisins

Preheat the oven to 350 degrees F. Place the water in a medium bowl, stir in the 2 tablespoons flaxseed meal, and let sit for 5 minutes. Place 16 fluted muffin liners in 2 muffin tins.

Add the shredded apples, milk, sweetener, and vanilla to the flaxseed mixture and stir to blend.

Place the flour, remaining ¾ cup flaxseed meal, oat bran, cinnamon, and baking powder in a large bowl, and whisk to combine. Add the milk mixture and stir with a spoon until blended, then add the raisins and stir to combine.

Fill the prepared muffin cups ¾ full and bake for 15 to 20 minutes, or until a paring knife inserted in a muffin has moist crumbs clinging to it. (We like our muffins moist, so we bake them for the shorter amount of time.) Let the muffins cool briefly in the tins, then remove to a wire rack to cool completely.

NO-BAKE peanut butter treats

YIELD: 12 TO 14 TREATS

These are a kid-friendly snack, and an easy treat that kids can help make. A little sticky, but fun!

¾ cup wheat germ

½ cup creamy unsalted dry roasted peanut butter

¼ cup raisins

2 tablespoons nutritional yeast

2 tablespoons liquid sweetener of your choice

¾ cup puffed wheat

Place the wheat germ, peanut butter, raisins, nutritional yeast, and sweetener in a medium bowl and stir to combine. Stir in the puffed wheat. Wet your hands with cold water, pick up teaspoon-sized clumps of the mixture and roll between your palms to form small balls.

VARIATION

Substitute another nut butter, such as almond or cashew butter, for the peanut butter.

GOLDEN **Pumpkin Muffins**

Pumpkin is a super source of potassium, which helps one think clearly (we should have eaten more of this when we were dating!), and has beta carotene, which contributes to healthy-looking skin.

¼ cup warm water

1 tablespoon flaxseed meal

½ cup dairy or nondairy milk

½ cup liquid sweetener of your choice

⅔ cup pumpkin purée, canned or freshly cooked

¼ cup canola oil

1¾ cups whole-wheat pastry flour

¼ cup cornmeal

1 teaspoon baking powder

1 teaspoon ground cinnamon

1 teaspoon ground allspice

1 teaspoon ground nutmeg

½ cup raisins

½ cup chopped pecans (optional)

Preheat the oven to 350 degrees F. Place the water in a large bowl, stir in the flaxseed meal, and let sit for 5 minutes. Line a muffin tin with fluted paper liners.

Add the milk, sweetener, pumpkin, and oil to the flaxseed mixture and stir to blend. Whisk together the flour, cornmeal, baking powder, and spices in a separate bowl, then stir the dry ingredients into the pumpkin mixture. Add the raisins and pecans (if using) and stir to blend.

Spoon the batter into the muffin cups. Bake for 20 minutes, or until a knife inserted in the center of a muffin comes out clean. Let the muffins cool briefly in the tin, then remove to a wire rack to cool completely.

banana tofu CUSTARD

YIELD: 2 SERVINGS

This great vegan breakfast treat filled with high-quality protein also makes a great dessert.

8 ounces firm tofu

2 ripe bananas

3 tablespoons thawed, unsweetened apple juice concentrate or 3 table-spoons liquid sweetener of your choice

2 tablespoons unsweetened shredded coconut

1 tablespoon canola oil

1 teaspoon vanilla extract

Process the tofu, bananas, apple juice concentrate, shredded coconut, oil, and vanilla in a blender until completely smooth. Pour the mixture into 2 custard cups and chill overnight.

CAROB **fudge balls**

Sometimes it is fun to have a no-bake, quick, cold treat in the refrigerator. These confections are great on-the-go snacks, high in potassium and riboflavin. Some people enjoy substituting carob in their diet instead of chocolate because chocolate contains caffeine, theobromine and oxalic acid.

3 tablespoons liquid sweetener of your choice

1 cup warm water

2 cups dry roasted, unsalted sunflower seeds

¾ cup carob powder

½ cup diced pitted dates

1 tablespoon vanilla extract

1 teaspoon ground cinnamon

½ cup unsweetened shredded coconut (optional)

Dissolve the sweetener in the water in a large bowl. Process the sunflower seeds in a blender until they become a powdery meal. Add the sunflower seed meal, carob powder, dates, vanilla, and cinnamon to the sweetened water and stir well to combine. Roll the mixture into bite-size balls, then roll the balls in the coconut (if using). Refrigerate for at least 2 hours.

corn bread DELIGHT

The millet adds a slight crunch to this delicious bread.

½ cup warm water

2 tablespoons flaxseed meal

2 cups corn kernels, fresh or frozen

1½ cups whole-wheat or unbleached pastry flour

1 cup cornmeal

¼ cup millet (optional)

1 tablespoon baking powder

1¼ cups dairy or nondairy milk

½ cup liquid sweetener of your choice

⅓ cup canola oil

Preheat the oven to 350 degrees F. Place the water in a medium bowl, stir in the flaxseed meal, and let sit for 5 minutes. Oil a 9 x 5-inch loaf pan.

Place the corn kernels, flour, cornmeal, millet (if using), and baking powder in a large bowl and stir until well combined. Add the milk, sweetener, and oil to the flax mixture and whisk to blend, then stir the liquid ingredients into the dry ingredients. Place the batter in the prepared loaf pan and bake for 30 minutes, or until a knife inserted in the center of the loaf comes out clean. Let the bread cool in the pan for 10 minutes, then turn out onto a wire rack and cool completely.

VARIATIONS

Mexican Corn Bread Delight. To give the bread a Mexican flair, add ½ cup diced onions, ⅓ cup diced red bell pepper and ½ cup shredded Monterey Jack or nondairy Monterey Jack–style cheese after adding the dry ingredients.

Delightful Corn Muffins. To make corn muffins, spoon the mixture into approximately 14 paper-lined muffin cups and bake for 20 minutes, or until a knife inserted in one of the muffins comes out clean. Let the muffins cool briefly in the tins, then remove to a wire rack to cool completely.

CRANBERRY **orange bread**

YIELD: 2 LOAVES

Cranberries are members of the blueberry family and are abundant during the months of October through December. Their bright red color adds a festive look to meals. Cranberries are rich in vitamin C and fiber.

¾ cup warm water

3 tablespoons flaxseed meal

Grated zest and juice of 2 oranges

1½ cups liquid sweetener of your choice

1 cup water

4 cups whole-wheat pastry flour

2 teaspoons baking powder

8 ounces cranberries, chopped or sliced (2 cups)

¾ cup walnuts, chopped

½ cup raisins

Preheat the oven to 350 degrees F. Place the ¾ cup warm water in a large bowl, stir in the flaxseed meal, and let sit for 5 minutes. Oil two 9 x 5-inch loaf pans.

Add the orange zest and juice, liquid sweetener, and 1 cup water to the flaxseed mixture and stir to blend. Whisk the flour and baking powder together in a medium bowl, then stir into the liquid ingredients, followed by the cranberries, nuts, and raisins. Stir just to incorporate. Divide the batter into the prepared pans. Bake for one hour, or until a paring knife inserted in the center of the loaf comes out clean. Let the bread cool in the pans for 10 minutes, then turn out onto a wire rack and cool completely.

BEACH **banana bread**

YIELD: ONE 9-INCH LOAF

We prefer moist breads and muffins and this is wonderfully moist bread. Look for ripe organic bananas with firm yellow skin and some dark spots.

¼ cup warm water

1 tablespoon flaxseed meal

3 ripe bananas, mashed

1 cup dairy or nondairy milk

½ cup liquid sweetener of your choice

⅓ cup canola oil

1½ cups whole-wheat pastry flour

1 cup rolled oats

1 cup oat bran

1 tablespoon baking powder

1 teaspoon ground cinnamon

½ teaspoon ground nutmeg

1 cup raisins

½ cup walnuts (optional)

Preheat the oven to 350 degrees F. Pour the water into a large bowl, add the flaxseed meal, and let sit for 5 minutes. Oil a 9 x 5-inch loaf pan.

Add the bananas, milk, sweetener, and oil to the flaxseed mixture, and stir until well combined. Whisk the flour, oats, oat bran, baking powder, cinnamon, and nutmeg in a medium bowl. Add the dry ingredients to the banana mixture and stir to incorporate, then stir in the raisins and walnuts (if using). Spoon the mixture into the prepared pan. Bake for 1 hour, or until the bread turns light golden brown. Let the bread cool in the pan for 10 minutes, then turn out onto a wire rack and cool completely.

SUNSATIONAL **cinnamon peaches**

YIELD: 1 TO 2 SERVINGS

This recipe is a real crowd pleaser. It is best with fresh peaches that are in season.

2 large, ripe peaches, sliced

½ cup water

1 tablespoon fresh lemon juice

1 tablespoon liquid sweetener of your choice

1 teaspoon ground ginger

1 teaspoon ground cinnamon

2 tablespoons raisins

Pinch ground nutmeg

Preheat the oven to 350 degrees F.
Place the peaches in a small baking dish. Whisk together the water, lemon juice, sweetener, ginger, and cinnamon in a small bowl, then stir in the raisins. Pour the mixture over the peaches. Sprinkle with the nutmeg and bake for 10 to 15 minutes or until the peaches become soft.

apple oat FLOAT

YIELD: 1 SERVING

This is a quick dairy-free breakfast or snack.

1¼ cups oat ring cereal (similar to Cheerios)

2 tablespoons walnuts, chopped fine

1 tablespoon raisins

1 tablespoon flaxseed meal

½ cup apple juice, cold

Place the cereal, nuts, raisins, and flaxseed in a bowl and add the apple juice.

VARIATIONS

Use puffed corn, wheat, or rice cereal in place of the oat rings.

great GRANOLA

The key to a great granola is to check on it while it is baking and stir the ingredients with a butter knife. Of course you need to be careful not to burn yourself.

⅔ cup canola oil

½ cup liquid sweetener of your choice

5 cups rolled oats

2½ cups chopped walnuts or pecans

2 cups unsweetened shredded or shaved coconut

1 cup raw sunflower seeds

1 cup oat bran

½ cup raisins

2 tablespoons flaxseed meal or flaxseeds

1 tablespoon pure vanilla extract

1 teaspoon ground cinnamon

Preheat the oven to 350 degrees F. Place the oil and sweetener in a large saucepan and warm over medium heat. Remove from the heat and stir in the oats, walnuts, coconut, sunflower seeds, oat bran, raisins, flaxseed meal, vanilla, and cinnamon. Mix well, then spread the mixture over a baking sheet and bake for 15 minutes, stirring with a butter knife occasionally. Store in a cool, dry place; keeps for up to one week, or store in quart-sized zipper-lock freezer bags for up to 3 months.

DEVRA'S **date bars**

YIELD: 12 BARS

The sweetness of pure dates is undeniable, just like our mother, Devra. Dates are a great source of fiber and a terrific energy food.

2 cups rolled oats

1 cup whole-wheat pastry flour

½ cup nonhydrogenated vegan margarine

8 ounces dates, pitted and chopped fine

2 tablespoons liquid sweetener of your choice

2 tablespoons fresh lemon juice

Preheat the oven to 350 degrees F.

Place the oats and flour in a large bowl and stir to combine. Add the margarine and mold the mixture with your hands until it forms a firm dough. Divide it in half and press half of it into a 7-inch square pan. Mix the dates, sweetener, and lemon juice in a large bowl and spread the mixture over the dough in the pan. Crumble the remaining dough over the date mixture. Bake for 30 minutes, or until the bars are light golden brown.

VARIATIONS

Apricot, Fig, or Blueberry Bars. Replace the dates with dried apricots or figs, or a cup of fresh blueberries.

Sunflower Date Bars. Add ½ cup dry-roasted sunflower seeds to the oats and flour for extra protein and crunch.

wholesome buttermilk PANCAKES

YIELD: 12 PANCAKES

Pancakes are fun to make with kids. Not only are oats a good source of protein and dietary fiber, they also reduce serum cholesterol levels. Fresh blueberries, strawberries or sliced bananas make a great topping for these whole-grain pancakes.

¼ cup warm water

1 tablespoon flaxseed meal

¾ cup buttermilk or rice, soy, or almond milk

1 tablespoon liquid sweetener of your choice

1 tablespoon canola oil

1 tablespoon vanilla extract

1 cup whole-wheat pastry flour

¼ cup oat flour

1 teaspoon baking powder

Place the water in a large bowl, stir in the flaxseed meal, and let sit for 5 minutes. Add the buttermilk, sweetener, oil, and vanilla to the flaxseed mixture and stir until well combined. Whisk the whole-wheat flour, oat flour, and baking powder together in a separate bowl, then stir in. Heat a large skillet or griddle until moderately hot and oil it lightly. For each pancake, pour about 2 heaping tablespoons of batter onto the hot pan. Cook each pancake until bubbles appear on the top, then flip and cook until the other side is a golden color. Serve with pure maple syrup.

PIE **crust**

YIELD: DOUGH FOR ONE 9-INCH 2-CRUST PIE

Pie crust can be made beforehand and stored in the refrigerator for up to a week, or in the freezer for up to six weeks.

2 cups whole-wheat pastry flour

¾ cup nonhydrogenated vegan margarine, softened, or canola oil

¼ cup ice water

1 tablespoon fresh lemon juice

Place the flour in a large mixing bowl. Use a fork or pastry blender to cut the margarine into the flour until the mixture consists of pea-size chunks. Stir in the ice water and lemon juice. Divide the dough in half and mold each half into a ball, then flatten the balls into disks. Use immediately or wrap the disks in plastic wrap and refrigerate.

yummy APPLE PIE

Shari's twin sons and husband ask for this pie on their birthdays!

Pie Crust (page 76)

6 medium green apples, peeled, cored and thinly sliced, about 5 cups

½ cup sweetener of your choice

½ cup raisins (optional)

3 tablespoons whole-wheat pastry flour

1 teaspoon vanilla extract

1 teaspoon ground cinnamon

½ teaspoon ground nutmeg

2 tablespoons nonhydrogenated vegan margarine, cut in small pieces

Preheat the oven to 350 degrees F.

Roll one disk of pie dough between two sheets of waxed paper until about ⅛ inch thick, and place it in a 9-inch pie plate. Bake the bottom crust for about 15 minutes. While the crust bakes, combine the apples, sweetener, raisins (if using), flour, vanilla, cinnamon, and nutmeg in a large bowl. Add the apple filling to the hot crust and dot the top of the filling with the margarine. Roll out the second disk of dough and place it on top of the filling. Crimp the edges to seal and poke holes in the top crust for the pie to "breathe." Bake for 45 minutes, or until the crust is golden brown and the juices are bubbling. Let cool before serving.

Note: Sometimes the edges of the crust become brown before the pie is done. To prevent this, place aluminum foil over the sides after the pie has baked for 20 minutes.

BLUEBERRY **bliss pie**

YIELD: ONE 9-INCH PIE

Blueberries are known for their cancer-preventing antioxidants and high vitamin C content. This pie tastes great topped with a scoop of dairy or nondairy vanilla ice cream.

Pie Crust (page 76)

5 cups blueberries, fresh or frozen

1 cup liquid sweetener of your choice

¼ cup fresh lemon juice, from 2 lemons

⅓ cup whole-wheat pastry flour or oat flour

1 teaspoon ground cinnamon

1 tablespoon nonhydrogenated vegan margarine, softened

Preheat the oven to 350 degrees F.

Roll one disk of pie dough between two sheets of waxed paper until about ⅛ inch thick, and place it in a 9-inch pie plate. Combine all the filling ingredients, except the margarine, in a large bowl and pour into the bottom crust. Dot the surface of the filling with the margarine. Roll out the second disk of dough and place it on top of the filling. Crimp the edges to seal and poke holes in the top crust for the pie to "breathe." Bake for 45 minutes, or until the crust is golden brown and the juices are bubbling. Let cool and serve with vanilla soy or rice cream.

Note: Sometimes the edges of the crust become brown before the pie is done. To prevent this, place aluminum foil over the sides after the pie has baked for 20 minutes.

pleasant PUMPKIN PIE

This low-fat version of a traditional pumpkin pie tastes creamy and rich.

Pie Crust (page 76)

1 can (15 ounces) pumpkin purée

14 ounces firm tofu

½ cup plus 2 tablespoons liquid sweetener of your choice

⅓ cup canola oil

½ teaspoon ground ginger

1 tablespoon ground cinnamon

1 teaspoon vanilla extract

1 teaspoon ground nutmeg

¼ teaspoon ground cloves

Preheat the oven to 350 degrees F.
Roll one disk of pie dough between 2 sheets of waxed paper until about ⅛ inch thick, and place it in a 9-inch pie plate. (Wrap and refrigerate or freeze the other disk of dough for later use.) Place all the filling ingredients in a blender and purée until smooth. Pour into the pie shell and bake for 40 to 50 minutes, or until the filling is set but just slightly wobbly. Let cool and place in the refrigerator overnight.

THE BEST peanut butter cream pie

YIELD: ONE 9-INCH PIE

This pie is so good and so easy to make. It tastes great frozen. It just melts in your mouth!

1 cup natural unsalted smooth peanut butter

1 box (8 ounces) low-fat dairy or nondairy cream cheese

14 ounces firm tofu or 1 cup dairy or nondairy whipping cream

½ cup sweetener of your choice

1 teaspoon vanilla extract

1 Graham Cracker Pie Crust (optional; page 81)

Place all the filling ingredients in a blender and blend until smooth. Pour into the graham cracker crust (if using) or directly into a pie pan and refrigerate overnight. If you don't use a crust, place the pie in the freezer overnight and then slice it into pieces when you want them. It's like eating peanut butter ice cream!

graham cracker PIE CRUST

Adding diced nuts to the graham crackers provides protein and a delicious twist to a traditional graham cracker crust.

10 whole graham crackers

3 tablespoons canola oil

3 tablespoons pure maple syrup

Preheat the oven to 350 degrees F.

Break up the graham crackers, place them in a food processor, and process them to fine crumbs. Transfer to a medium bowl and add the canola oil and maple syrup. Turn the mixture into a 9-inch pie pan and press into the bottom and up the sides to form an even crust. Bake for 10 minutes or until light golden brown.

Note: We use honey-sweetened graham crackers for the crust.

VARIATION

Cookie Crumb Crust. Substitute cookie crumbs for the graham cracker crumbs. Place 12 medium size cookies (approximately 2 inches in diameter) in a zipper-lock bag and squeeze until the cookies are crumbled. Add ½ cup of finely chopped nuts, if desired, before mixing with the oil and maple syrup.

Additional Breakfast Hints

Fresh fruits are our favorite breakfast. We like to have them with yogurt and cereal. When choosing fresh fruit for breakfast, try to buy fruit that's in season locally. For example, during the month of June, plums come into season and they are delightful for breakfast. In July, raspberries are in season and they are wonderful on cereal or alone. (Did you know raspberries are from the rose family? They are our favorite "rose.") At the end of this book, we've included a monthly calendar for buying fresh, in-season produce; see page 139. Please refer to it when choosing fresh fruit for breakfast. Many grocery stores have certain fruits all year long because they import them from other countries. Unfortunately, imported produce is often heavily sprayed with chemicals. We buy domestic, preferably organic, produce.

Whenever you are eating cereal with yogurt or milk (or rice, soy or almond milk), you can boost your nutrition by adding flaxseed meal, oat bran and/or nutritional yeast. Flaxseeds are high in omega 3-fatty acids, lignans (plant estrogens which have an antioxidant effect), and both insoluble and soluble fiber. Oat bran is another excellent source of soluble fiber, which lowers cholesterol. Nutritional yeast is full of B vitamins, which help convert food into energy. Of course all these added ingredients can be used in a breakfast smoothie, too.

Moderate Lunches

9

Our largest meal of the day occurs at lunch, allowing ample time for digestion before going to bed at night. Take a moment to be grateful for the fresh foods you have to eat, chew your food thoroughly, and enjoy your meals. It's fun to "m-m-m" and "ahh" during a meal. Appreciate the way your food tastes, and embrace the joy of eating.

LUNCHES

anacapa ANTIPASTO

A terrific munch for lunch! We offer two versions of this salad.

GROUP 1: *Traditional Vegetables*

2 heads cauliflower, chopped (about
6 cups)

1 large bunch broccoli, chopped
(about 4 cups)

4 medium carrots, diced (about
2 cups)

1 large zucchini, diced (about
2 cups)

1 medium red bell pepper, seeded
and chopped (about ¾ cup)

GROUP 2: *Italian vegetables*

1 pound cherry tomatoes

8 ounces white mushrooms, sliced
thick (about 1 cup)

1 medium red bell pepper, seeded
and chopped (about ¾ cup)

2 green onions, chopped

1 can (6 ounces) sliced black olives,
drained, or pitted Greek olives

1 can (6 ounces) artichoke hearts,
drained and quartered

DRESSING

½ cup tomato-based chili sauce

¼ cup fresh lemon juice, from
2 lemons

¼ cup red wine vinegar

2 tablespoons extra-virgin olive oil

4 garlic cloves, minced

1 teaspoon dried basil

1 teaspoon dried oregano

½ teaspoon dry mustard

Pinch dried or chopped fresh parsley

Place all the vegetables from Group 1 or Group 2 in a large bowl. Combine the dressing ingredients in a small saucepan and bring to a boil. Immediately pour the hot dressing over the vegetables. Toss gently and place in the refrigerator. Chill for a few hours and serve cold.

APPLESAUCE rice cake sandwiches

We love sandwiches made on whole-grain breads, but sometimes we like to use rice cakes for variety.

1 cup unsweetened applesauce

1 apple, peeled and grated

½ cup raisins

½ cup finely chopped walnuts

1 teaspoon ground cinnamon

1 teaspoon ground nutmeg

Smooth unsalted dry roasted or raw almond butter

6 rice cakes

Mix the applesauce, grated apple, raisins, walnuts, cinnamon, and nutmeg in a medium bowl. Spread almond butter on 3 of the rice cakes, then spoon 2 tablespoons of the applesauce mixture over the almond butter. Place the remaining 3 rice cakes on top to form sandwiches.

VARIATIONS

Try peanut butter or cashew butter instead of the almond butter.

Sprinkle some dairy or nondairy shredded cheese on top of the applesauce mixture (do not top with the remaining rice cakes). Place the rice cakes in a toaster oven or under a broiler and heat until the cheese is melted and bubbly.

SEASIDE **shell salad**

Preparing this salad the night before you eat it is worth it. On a hot summer day it's great to just pull this salad out of the refrigerator and toss it over a bed of greens or eat it right out of the bowl.

8 ounces small pasta shells

⅓ cup apple cider vinegar

4 tablespoons extra-virgin olive oil

½ cup sliced black olives

2 green onions, sliced thin

8 ounces cherry tomatoes, halved (about 1 cup)

½ cup fresh shelled green peas

2 garlic cloves, minced

2 teaspoons dried Italian herb blend (basil, parsley, and oregano flakes)

1 teaspoon freshly ground black pepper

1 small head butter lettuce, washed and leaves separated (optional)

½ cup pine nuts

Freshly grated Parmesan cheese or nondairy Parmesan-style cheese

Cook the pasta according to the package directions, then drain and rinse with cold water. Place the pasta in a large bowl. Stir the vinegar and oil together in a glass, pour the mixture over the cold pasta, and stir. Add the olives, green onions, tomatoes, peas, garlic, herbs, and pepper; toss to combine. Cover the bowl with plastic wrap and refrigerate at least 2 hours or overnight. To serve, arrange lettuce leaves (if using) on a platter or individual plates, spoon the pasta salad on top, and sprinkle with the pine nuts and Parmesan.

Note: You can use any type of chunky pasta, such as penne or rotelle, in this dish.

TEMPTING TEMPEH **with soba noodles**

YIELD: 4 SERVINGS

Soba noodles are Japanese noodles made with buckwheat. Tempeh, made from fermented soybeans, is filled with soy isoflavones, known to strengthen bones, ease menopausal symptoms, and reduce coronary heart disease. Together, the noodles and tempeh make a fiber-rich, protein-packed meal.

3 tablespoons tamari (soy sauce)

3 tablespoons rice vinegar

2 tablespoons sesame oil

1 tablespoon liquid sweetener of your choice

2 teaspoons chili paste

2 garlic cloves, minced

8 ounces tempeh, cut in 1-inch cubes

8 ounces soba noodles or any spaghetti-type pasta

8 ounces sugar snap peas, rinsed and trimmed

½ cup diced red bell pepper

¼ cup sliced green onions

¼ cup chopped fresh cilantro

Bring 3 quarts of water to a boil in a large pot. Place the tamari, rice vinegar, sesame oil, sweetener, chili paste, and garlic in a large bowl and whisk to combine. Add the tempeh cubes and gently toss to coat all sides.

Cook the tempeh cubes in a large skillet over medium heat about 5 minutes, or until they turn light brown, stirring often. Return the cooked tempeh to the bowl.

Add the soba noodles to the boiling water and cook, uncovered, for 5 minutes or until almost al dente. Add the peas and bell pepper and cook for 1 minute more. Drain well and transfer the hot noodles, peas, and bell pepper to the tempeh-sauce mixture. Toss in the cilantro and green onions. Serve warm.

VARIATION

Sprinkle ½ cup slivered almonds over the noodles for added crunch.

EASTSIDE **enchiladas**

YIELD: 12 SERVINGS

These enchiladas are incredibly easy to make, yet good enough for company—we make them whenever we have guests coming to town. Even the meat eaters love them!

1 jar (16 ounces) salsa, plus ¼ cup for garnish

2 boxes (8 ounces each) dairy or nondairy cream cheese, softened

10 ounces Monterey Jack cheese or nondairy Monterey Jack–style cheese, shredded (2½ cups)

1 package (14 ounces) firm tofu, crumbled

1 can (3.8 ounces) sliced black olives, drained (about 1 cup)

1 bunch green onions, chopped

1 large red bell pepper, seeded and diced

1 celery stalk, diced

1 garlic clove, minced

12 no-lard flour tortillas

Preheat the oven to 350 degrees F.

Place the salsa, cream cheese, 2 cups of the shredded cheese, tofu, olives, green onions, bell pepper, celery, and garlic in a large bowl and stir to combine. Lay a tortilla on the counter, place a couple of large spoonfuls of filling in the center, and roll the tortilla around the filling. Place the filled tortilla in a 9 x 13-inch baking dish and repeat with the remaining tortillas and filling. Sprinkle the ¼ cup of salsa on top, and then sprinkle the remaining ½ cup shredded cheese on top of the enchiladas. Bake for 25 minutes or until the filling is hot and the cheese is browned and bubbling.

VARIATION

Eastside Bean Enchiladas. Replace the tofu with one 16-ounce can of pinto beans.

great grilled PORTOBELLOS

YIELD: 8 SERVINGS

Portobello mushrooms provide niacin, potassium and selenium and have a savory, meaty taste. Serve these mushrooms on their own as a side dish or on toasted buns for a delicious sandwich.

3 tablespoons extra-virgin olive oil

3 garlic cloves, minced

1 tablespoon fresh lemon juice

8 large portobello mushrooms, brushed clean and stems removed

1 tablespoon freshly grated Parmesan cheese or nondairy Parmesan-style cheese

1 tablespoon dried Italian herb blend (basil, parsley, and oregano flakes) or minced fresh basil

Light the grill. Place the olive oil in a small saucepan, add the garlic, and sauté briefly, until the garlic becomes fragrant. Remove from the heat and stir in the lemon juice. Brush the mushrooms all over with the garlic mixture and grill stem-side down over medium heat for about 8 minutes. Flip the mushrooms and cook stem-side up for another 8 minutes, or until they are browned and tender. Place them on a serving platter and sprinkle with the Parmesan and herbs. Serve immediately.

VARIATION

Great Sautéed Portobellos. If the weather's not right for grilling, you can make this dish on the stove. Heat the olive oil in a large skillet over medium heat, add the garlic, and sauté for a couple of minutes, then stir in the lemon juice. Place 4 of the mushrooms in the skillet, increase the heat slightly, and sauté for about 5 minutes, turning the mushrooms so that they cook on both sides, until they are tender. Remove the mushrooms to a serving platter and cover to keep warm while you repeat with the remaining mushrooms. Sprinkle the mushrooms with the Parmesan and herbs and serve.

guacamole MJELDE

YIELD: 1 CUP

Avocados are a rich fruit packed with nutrition. This guacamole is delicious on tortilla chips, rice cakes, crackers, a bed of lettuce, or all by itself.

3 large Hass avocados, mashed

½ cup salsa

1 tomato, diced fine

1 onion, diced fine

3 tablespoons fresh lemon juice

2 garlic cloves, minced

1 teaspoon garlic powder

1 teaspoon sea salt (optional)

Place all the ingredients into a large bowl and stir until well combined. Serve immediately or press plastic wrap directly on the surface to prevent browning and refrigerate.

EGG-CEPTIONAL **eggplant parmesan**

YIELD: 4 SERVINGS

Enjoy this baked, not fried, version of an Italian favorite!

1 large eggplant, peeled and sliced ½ inch thick

½ cup warm water

2 tablespoons flaxseed meal

½ cup plain dairy or nondairy yogurt

1 cup dry bread crumbs

1½ cups tomato sauce

1 cup sliced white mushrooms

1 can (3.8 ounces) sliced black olives, drained (about 1 cup)

2 garlic cloves, minced

2 teaspoons dried Italian herb blend (basil, parsley, and oregano flakes)

4 ounces mozzarella cheese or nondairy mozzarella-style cheese, shredded (1 cup)

½ cup freshly grated Parmesan cheese or nondairy Parmesan-style cheese

Preheat the oven to 350 degrees F.

Place the sliced eggplant in a large bowl, add enough warm water to cover, and let the slices soak for 20 minutes. Drain the eggplant, then press each slice between paper towels to remove any excess liquid.

While the eggplant soaks, place the ½ cup warm water in a medium bowl, stir in the flaxseed meal, and let sit for 5 minutes. Stir in the yogurt. Dip the eggplant slices into this mixture and then sprinkle each side with breadcrumbs. Place the breaded slices into a 9 x 13-inch pan.

Place the tomato sauce, mushrooms, olives, garlic, and herbs in a medium bowl and stir to blend. Spread evenly over the eggplant slices. Distribute the shredded cheese over the sauce and sprinkle with the Parmesan. Bake for 45 minutes, or until the tomato sauce is bubbling and the cheese is lightly browned. Serve immediately.

Note: When buying bread crumbs, read labels and avoid brands with preservatives, additives and sugars. You can also make your own bread crumbs from stale bread. Just cut slices of bread in small squares and toast the bread in a toaster oven at 350 degrees F for 10 minutes, or until the bread is slightly browned.

TANNER'S **tasty tostadas**

YIELD: 6 SERVINGS

This is an easy and quick meal.

6 corn tortillas

1 can (16 ounces) vegetarian refried beans or 1 cup cooked pinto beans

2 cups cooked brown rice

4 ounces cheddar cheese or nondairy cheddar-style cheese, shredded (1½ cups)

2 large tomatoes, diced

1 small head romaine lettuce, shredded

3 green onions, chopped fine

2 ripe Hass avocados, sliced

1 can (6 ounces) sliced black olives, drained

¼ cup medium-heat salsa

½ cup dairy or nondairy sour cream

½ cup Guacamole Mjelde (page 90)

Preheat the oven to 350 degrees F.
Place the corn tortillas on a baking sheet and bake for 10 minutes or until crisp. Spread a heaping spoonful of beans on each crisp tortilla, then add a spoonful of rice. Sprinkle each tortilla with cheese and bake for another 5 minutes. Place the tomatoes, lettuce, onions, avocados, olives, salsa, sour cream, and guacamole in individual bowls, and serve the tostadas, letting each person choose their own toppings.

protein-packed POCKET

YIELD: 1 SERVING

Pocket breads are fun sandwich breads.

¼ cup firm tofu, crumbled (see note)

½ cup diced red bell pepper

½ cup diced tomato

1 green onion, diced

1 tablespoon vegan mayonnaise

1 whole-wheat pocket bread (pita), cut in half

1 ounce dry roasted almonds, chopped (about ¼ cup)

½ cup alfalfa sprouts

Stir the tofu, pepper, tomato, green onion, and mayonnaise together in a medium bowl. Stuff the mixture into both halves of the pocket bread and sprinkle with the almonds and sprouts.

Note: Marinated tofu is available in many different savory flavors and can be found in the deli or refrigerated section of natural foods stores.

ranch style FETTUCCINE

YIELD: 4 SERVINGS

This is a colorful dish filled with nutrition.

12 ounces fettuccine

¼ cup nonhydrogenated vegan margarine or extra-virgin olive oil

1 medium red bell pepper, seeded and diced

8 white mushrooms, sliced thin

1 carrot, diced

¼ cup sliced green onions

2 garlic cloves, minced

½ cup fresh or thawed frozen green peas

½ teaspoon dried basil

½ teaspoon dried parsley

½ teaspoon freshly ground black pepper

½ cup freshly grated Parmesan cheese or nondairy Parmesan-style cheese

Cook the fettuccine according to the package directions. While the fettuccine is cooking, heat the margarine in a large skillet. Add the bell pepper, mushrooms, carrot, onions, and garlic and cook, stirring, about 5 minutes, or until the vegetables are softened and lightly browned. Add the peas, basil, parsley, and black pepper. Drain the fettuccine, add it to the skillet and stir gently. Top with the Parmesan and serve immediately.

IRRESISTIBLE lasagne roll-ups

YIELD: 5 SERVINGS

This is a quick version of traditional lasagne.

10 plain or spinach lasagne noodles, cooked according to package directions

¼ cup warm water

1 tablespoon flaxseed meal

1 large bunch spinach, chopped fine (about 2½ cups)

1 cup low-fat dairy or nondairy cottage cheese (ricotta cheese can be substituted)

¼ cup freshly grated Parmesan cheese or nondairy Parmesan-style cheese, plus extra for sprinkling

¼ cup diced yellow onion

2 garlic cloves, minced

½ teaspoon ground nutmeg

½ teaspoon fennel seed

3 cups tomato sauce

Preheat the oven to 350 degrees F.

Place the water in a large bowl, stir in the flaxseed meal, and let sit for 5 minutes. Add the spinach, cottage cheese, Parmesan, onion, garlic, nutmeg, and fennel, and stir the ingredients together with a large spoon. Spread a couple of spoonfuls of the filling onto each cooked lasagne noodle and roll up the noodles carefully. Place each roll on end in a 9 x 13-inch casserole dish. Cover with the tomato sauce and extra Parmesan. Bake for 25 minutes or until the sauce starts to bubble. Serve immediately.

SATISFYING **stuffed bell peppers**

YIELD: 2 SERVINGS

Tired of getting your vitamin C boost from orange juice? Try bell peppers! Peppers contain lots of potassium and beta carotene, too.

¼ cup warm water

1 tablespoon flaxseed meal

2 large red, green, or yellow bell peppers

14 ounces firm tofu, crumbled

1 cup cooked brown or wild rice

½ cup freshly grated Parmesan cheese or nondairy Parmesan-style cheese, plus extra for sprinkling

½ yellow onion, diced

1 tablespoon toasted wheat germ

1 tablespoon tamari

1 garlic clove, minced

1 teaspoon dried parsley

½ teaspoon dried oregano

½ teaspoon dried rosemary

1 teaspoon paprika

Preheat the oven to 350 degrees F.

Place the water in a medium bowl, stir in the flaxseed meal, and let sit for 5 minutes. Slice the tops off the bell peppers and scoop out the seeds. Add the tofu, rice, ½ cup of the Parmesan, the onion, wheat germ, tamari, garlic, parsley, oregano, and rosemary to the bowl with the flaxseed mixture and stir to combine. Stuff the bell peppers with the mixture; sprinkle additional Parmesan and the paprika on top. Place the peppers upright in a small pan (such as an 8 x 4-inch loaf pan) and bake for 20 minutes. Serve immediately.

VARIATION

Replace the tofu with 1½ cups dairy or nondairy cottage cheese.

NUTTY **non-meat loaf**

This vegetarian version of the classic comfort food cuts the calories and fat, not the flavor. It makes a protein-packed meal that can be prepared ahead of time and stored in the refrigerator for up to a week. Serve it hot or cold crumbled on salads or sliced in sandwiches.

½ cup warm water

2 tablespoons flaxseed meal

3 cups cooked brown rice (see note)

2 ounces cheddar cheese or nondairy cheddar-style cheese, shredded (about ½ cup)

½ cup finely chopped walnuts

½ cup toasted sunflower seeds

1 onion, chopped (about ½ cup)

1 carrot, grated (about ½ cup)

¼ cup minced fresh parsley

¼ cup sunflower oil

¼ cup whole-wheat flour

1 garlic clove, minced

½ teaspoon dried thyme

½ teaspoon dried basil

½ teaspoon dried oregano

½ teaspoon dried rosemary

Preheat the oven to 350 degrees F. Lightly oil a 9 x 5-inch loaf pan.

Place the warm water in a large bowl, stir in the flaxseed mixture and let sit for 5 minutes. Add the rice, cheese, walnuts, sunflower seeds, onion, carrot, parsley, oil, flour, garlic, thyme, basil, oregano, and rosemary, and stir to combine thoroughly. Place the mixture in the prepared pan. Cover the pan with aluminum foil and bake for 45 minutes. Serve immediately.

Note: To make 3 cups brown rice, bring 2 cups water to a boil in a medium saucepan, add 1 cup brown rice, cover, reduce heat, and simmer 35 to 45 minutes, or until all the water is absorbed.

SURF'S UP **tofu salad sandwich**

YIELD: 2 SERVINGS

Tofu is high in protein and easily digested. It's also tremendously versatile because it absorbs flavors from the ingredients mixed with it.

8 ounces firm tofu, drained

2 kosher pickles, diced

1 celery stalk, diced

¼ cup vegan mayonnaise

½ teaspoon mustard

¼ teaspoon minced onion

¼ teaspoon turmeric

4 slices whole-grain bread

½ cucumber, sliced (optional)

1 large tomato, sliced (optional)

Crumble the tofu into a medium bowl and mash into small pieces with a fork. Add the pickles, celery, mayonnaise, mustard, onion, and turmeric to the tofu and mix well. Spread on the bread slices and top with cucumber slices and tomato slices (if using).

Note: The tofu mixture can be spread on crackers, or place a scoop on top of any of your favorite salads. This salad can be made ahead of time and stored in the refrigerator in an airtight container for up to week.

sunset sun BURGERS

These vegetarian burgers are delicious and nutritious! We like to serve them with the works....cheese, pickles, ketchup, mayonnaise, tomatoes and lettuce.

½ cup warm water

2 tablespoons flaxseed meal

1½ cups ground dry roasted sunflower seeds or 1 cup sunflower seeds and ½ cup dry roasted peanuts

1 carrot, grated (about ½ cup)

1 celery stalk, diced (about ½ cup)

1 onion, diced

½ red bell pepper, diced

2 tablespoons minced fresh parsley

2 tablespoons tamari

2 tablespoons nutritional yeast

2 tablespoons whole-wheat flour or oat flour

1 teaspoon dried basil

1 teaspoon garlic powder

4 whole-grain hamburger buns

Preheat the oven to 350 degrees F. Lightly oil a baking sheet. Place the warm water in a large bowl, stir in the flaxseed meal, and let sit for 5 minutes. Add the sunflower seeds, carrot, celery, onion, bell pepper, parsley, tamari, nutritional yeast, flour, basil, and garlic powder and mix until completely blended. Divide the mixture into 4 even portions and form each portion into a patty. Place the patties on the prepared sheet and bake for about 20 minutes, then flip the patties over and continue to bake for 20 more minutes. Serve the patties on the buns, accompanied with your favorite condiments.

MATTEA'S FAVORITE **pizza dough**

YIELD: DOUGH FOR 4 TO 6 INDIVIDUAL PIZZAS (SEE NOTE)

Our kids love to make pizza! This crust recipe is a big hit with everyone and is the base for a variety of great pizza toppings.

1¼ cups warm water

1 envelope (2¼ teaspoons) active dry yeast

1 tablespoon liquid sweetener of your choice

3 cups whole-wheat flour

2 tablespoons extra-virgin olive oil, plus extra for the bowl and baking sheets

1 tablespoon dried Italian herb blend (basil, parsley, and oregano flakes)

¼ cup cornmeal or flour for the counter

Pour the warm water into a large glass or ceramic mixing bowl. Sprinkle the yeast over the water and add the sweetener. Let the yeast mixture stand for 5 to 10 minutes or until bubbly.

Stir in the flour, oil, and herbs to make a soft dough. Sprinkle cornmeal or flour (or a combination) on the counter and knead the dough for about 5 minutes or until it appears smooth and satiny, adding more cornmeal or flour as necessary to prevent sticking.

Oil the bowl and return the dough to it. Cover with plastic wrap or a damp dish towel and place in a warm, draft-free place for about an hour or until the dough has doubled in volume. Oil 2 large baking sheets. Punch down the dough and divide it into 4 equal pieces, then shape each piece into a round. Place 2 dough rounds on each prepared baking sheet and pat into 6-inch circles, pinching the edges to form a raised rim.

Note: For thin-crust pizzas, divide the dough into 6 equal pieces and shape as above, placing 3 rounds on each baking sheet.

PIZZA **dough 2**

This is a lighter pizza dough; it uses enriched white flour instead of whole-wheat flour.

1¾ cups warm water

1 envelope (2¼ teaspoons) active dry yeast

1 tablespoon liquid sweetener of your choice

4 cups unbleached enriched all-purpose flour

2 tablespoons extra-virgin olive oil, plus extra for the bowl and baking sheets

½ teaspoon dried Italian herb blend (basil, parsley, and oregano flakes)

¼ cup cornmeal or flour for dusting the counter

Pour the warm water into a large glass or ceramic mixing bowl. Sprinkle the yeast over the water and add the sweetener. Let the mixture stand for 5 to 10 minutes or until bubbly.

Stir in the flour, oil, and herbs to make a soft dough. Sprinkle cornmeal or flour (or a combination) on the counter and knead the dough for about 5 minutes or until it appears smooth and satiny, adding more cornmeal or flour as necessary to prevent sticking.

Oil the bowl and return the dough to it. Cover with plastic wrap or a damp dish towel and place in a warm, draft-free place for about an hour or until the dough has doubled in volume. Oil 2 large baking sheets. Punch down the dough and divide it into 3 equal pieces, then shape each piece into a round. Place 2 dough rounds on one prepared baking sheet and 1 on the other sheet and pat into 9-inch circles, pinching the edges to form a raised rim.

Note: Although this dough is time-consuming to make, it stores well, so you can make it ahead of time and it's ready to roll out when you need it. After punching down the dough, place it in a well-sealed plastic bag and refrigerate it for up to 5 days.

GIOVANNA'S **italian classico pizzas**

YIELD: 3 MEDIUM PIZZAS

Our Italian grandmother, Giovanna, is the inspiration for this pizza. She and her mother, Alma, had an amazing vegetable garden; the fresh vegetables they picked during the day would top that night's pizza.

Mattea's Favorite Pizza Dough (page 100) **or Pizza Dough 2** (page 101)

1 cup pizza sauce

1 yellow onion, diced

2 garlic cloves, minced

1 cup sliced white mushrooms

⅓ cup sliced black olives

1 tablespoon chopped fresh parsley

½ cup shredded mozzarella cheese or nondairy mozzarella-style cheese

¼ cup freshly grated Parmesan cheese or nondairy Parmesan-style cheese

Preheat the oven to 350 degrees F. Following the directions in the pizza dough recipe, pat the dough out into circles on baking sheets.

Use a tablespoon to spoon the amount of tomato sauce desired in the middle of the flattened pizza dough. Place the onion, garlic, mushrooms, olives, and parsley on top of the tomato sauce. Sprinkle the cheeses on top and bake for about 15 minutes, or until the cheese has melted and the crust is golden brown. Serve immediately.

Note: We like Asiago cheese in this pizza too; you can substitute it for the Parmesan.

fiesta combo PIZZAS

YIELD: 3 MEDIUM PIZZAS

Mexican food is festive and flavorful. Cilantro (also known as fresh coriander leaves) adds flair to this pizza. If you're daring like Shari, go for hot salsa, and if you're conservative like Judi, go for mild salsa.

Mattea's Favorite Pizza Dough (page 100) **or Pizza Dough 2** (page 101)

1 cup pizza sauce or salsa

1 can (6 ounces) diced green chilies

4 tomatoes, sliced

⅓ cup sliced black olives

⅓ cup corn kernels

3 green onions, chopped

2 tablespoons fresh cilantro

1 cup shredded mozzarella cheese or nondairy mozzarella-style cheese

Preheat the oven to 350 degrees F. Following the directions in the pizza dough recipe, pat the dough out into circles on baking sheets. Divide the tomato sauce evenly among the pizza crusts, then top with the tomatoes, olives, corn, green onions, and cilantro.

Sprinkle the cheese on last and bake for 10 minutes, or until the cheese is melted and the crust is a light golden brown. Serve immediately.

ASIAN-STYLE **pizzas**

YIELD: 3 MEDIUM PIZZAS

Crystallized ginger adds an unusual, but delicious, accent flavor to this pizza. Ginger is also a natural aid for digestion.

Mattea's Favorite Pizza Dough (page 100) **or Pizza Dough 2** (page 101)

¼ cup sesame oil

2 tablespoons minced crystallized ginger

1 tablespoon orange juice

4 tomatoes, sliced

¾ cup sliced water chestnuts

½ cup sliced snow peas

1 small onion, diced

¾ cup shredded mozzarella cheese or nondairy mozzarella-style cheese

Combine the oil, ginger, and orange juice in a large bowl, then add the tomatoes, water chestnuts, snow peas, and onion, and let the vegetables marinate for at least 1 hour. Preheat the oven to 350 degrees F. Following the directions in the pizza dough recipe, pat the dough out into circles on baking sheets. Divide the marinated vegetable mixture among the pizza crusts and sprinkle the cheese on top. Bake for 10 minutes, or until the cheese has melted and the crust is a light golden brown. Serve immediately.

SPINACH FLORENTINE **pizzas**

Spinach is high in vitamin K (important to maintaining bone health) and iron. Adding spinach to pizza, raviolis, and other foods is a tempting way to prepare it that children will enjoy.

Mattea's Favorite Pizza Dough (page 100) **or Pizza Dough 2** (page 101)

1 tablespoon flaxseed meal

¼ cup warm water

½ lemon

1 bunch spinach, stems removed

3 tablespoons extra-virgin olive oil

1 small red onion, sliced thin

1 cup tomato sauce

½ teaspoon ground nutmeg

1 cup shredded mozzarella cheese or nondairy mozzarella-style cheese

½ cup grated Gruyère cheese or nondairy Swiss-style cheese

Preheat the oven to 350 degrees F. Following the directions in the pizza dough recipe, pat the dough out into circles on baking sheets.

Stir the flaxseed meal into the warm water and let sit for 5 minutes. Fill a large bowl with cold water and squeeze the lemon half into the bowl. Wash the spinach leaves in the lemon water, then drain the spinach and pat dry with paper towels. Heat the oil in a large skillet over medium heat. Add the onion and sauté, stirring, until soft, then add the spinach and cook until the spinach wilts. Drain off any excess liquid. Divide the tomato sauce evenly among the pizza crusts and then place some of the spinach mixture on top of each. In a small bowl, beat the flaxseed mixture with the nutmeg and pour over the spinach. Top with both cheeses. Bake for 10 minutes, or until the cheese has melted and the crust is a light golden brown. Serve immediately.

VARIATIONS

The pizza crust recipes can be the foundation for many different toppings, so feel free to experiment. Some of our favorites include Gorgonzola cheese with sliced pears or pineapple with walnuts and raisins.

Light Dinners

We believe if you are going to eat at night, it better be light! Salads and soups are your best choices.

DINNERS

seaside CAESAR SALAD

YIELD: 4 SERVINGS

This Caesar salad is anchovy-free but filled with flavor.

¼ cup extra-virgin olive oil

2 tablespoons fresh lemon juice

2 garlic cloves, minced

½ teaspoon freshly ground black pepper

1 head romaine lettuce, washed and torn into small pieces

¾ cup natural croutons

1 tomato, chopped

¼ cup freshly grated Parmesan or Asiago cheese or nondairy Parmesan-style cheese

Place the olive oil, lemon juice, garlic, and black pepper in a blender and process to blend.

Place the lettuce in a large bowl, add the croutons, tomato, and Parmesan, then pour the dressing over the top and toss until the salad ingredients are coated.

VARIATION

Add pine nuts and vegetarian bacon bits.

CALIFORNIA **cool slaw**

YIELD: 3 SERVINGS

This delicious coleslaw is an easy side dish or it can be scooped into a whole-wheat pocket bread for a fun sandwich.

⅓ cup vegan mayonnaise

3 tablespoons fresh lemon juice

2 tablespoons plain dairy or nondairy yogurt (optional)

1 tablespoon liquid sweetener of your choice

½ teaspoon freshly ground black pepper

2½ cups shredded green cabbage

2 carrots, grated

2 celery stalks, diced

½ onion, diced

1 tablespoon raisins (optional)

Whisk the mayonnaise, lemon juice, yogurt, sweetener, and pepper together in a large bowl. Add the cabbage, carrots, celery, onion, and raisins (if using) and toss to coat the vegetables thoroughly. Place the coleslaw in an airtight container and refrigerate for at least 2 hours before eating.

EL CAPITAN **potato salad**

This potato salad is great for summer celebration meals, especially good for the Fourth of July!

6 red potatoes, scrubbed and cut in 1-inch cubes

3 pickles, diced

2 celery stalks, diced

6 green onions, chopped fine

¾ cup vegan mayonnaise

⅓ cup apple cider vinegar

2 tablespoons plain dairy or nondairy yogurt

1 teaspoon freshly ground black pepper

½ teaspoon celery seed

½ teaspoon paprika

Bring 2 quarts of water to a boil in a large saucepan, add the potatoes, and cook 10 to 15 minutes, or until tender. Drain the potatoes and place them in a large bowl, then add the pickles, celery and green onions. Whisk the mayonnaise, vinegar, yogurt, black pepper, celery seed and paprika together in a medium bowl, then pour over the potatoes and stir to coat. Place the salad in an airtight container and refrigerate for 2 hours before serving.

asian CUKE SALAD

Cucumbers are high in potassium and they add a terrific crunchy texture to salads.

1 long English hothouse cucumber or 2 large peeled cucumbers, sliced thin

20 sugar snap peas, trimmed and cut in thirds

½ cup thinly sliced white mushrooms

½ cup apple cider vinegar

¼ cup toasted sesame seeds, plus extra for garnish

2 tablespoons sesame oil

1 tablespoon liquid sweetener of your choice

1 tablespoon tamari

1 large tomato, sliced thin

Dried dill weed

Combine the cucumber, peas, and mushrooms in a large bowl. Add the vinegar, sesame seeds, sesame oil, sweetener, and tamari and toss to blend. Place the salad in an airtight container and refrigerate for at least 2 hours. Before serving, garnish the mixture with the tomato slices and sprinkle dill and extra sesame seeds over the top.

festival GREEK SALAD

This tasty salad is fun to serve with whole-wheat pita chips.

1 head romaine lettuce, washed and torn into pieces

½ head cauliflower, cleaned and separated into florets

½ large red pepper, seeded and diced

1 medium tomato, diced

½ medium cucumber, sliced

1 cup sliced Greek or Kalamata olives

8 ounces feta cheese, crumbled, or crumbled seasoned tofu

¾ cup plain dairy or nondairy yogurt

2 tablespoons vegan mayonnaise

1 tablespoon extra-virgin olive oil

2 tablespoons fresh lemon juice

1 garlic clove, minced

1 teaspoon freshly ground black pepper

Place the romaine lettuce in a large salad bowl. Mix the cauliflower, red pepper, tomato, cucumber, olives, and feta in a separate bowl, then add to the lettuce. Whisk the yogurt, mayonnaise, olive oil, lemon juice, garlic, and black pepper together in a small bowl. Toss with the vegetables and serve.

SNAPPY **pea salad**

This chilled salad is refreshing and nutritious.

1 head butter lettuce, torn into pieces

1 cup raw, shelled fresh English peas or thinly sliced sugar snap peas

1 cup raw cashews

1 ripe avocado, peeled and sliced

¼ cup cubed jícama

¼ cup sliced radishes

¼ cup cooked corn kernels

¼ cup cubed Monterey Jack cheese or nondairy Monterey Jack–style cheese

¾ cup Creamy Italian Dressing (page 118)

¼ cup vegetarian bacon bits

½ cup alfalfa sprouts

Combine the lettuce, peas, cashews, avocado, jícama, radishes, corn, and cheese in a large bowl. Cover and refrigerate for at least an hour. Just before serving, toss with the dressing and top with the vegetarian bacon bits and alfalfa sprouts.

IRWIN'S **waldorf salad**

YIELD: 4 SERVINGS

Our father, Irwin Zucker, is a fantastic father and an extremely energetic public relations man in Hollywood, California. He's "promotion in motion." One might say that the apple doesn't fall far from the tree, because we are very similar to our dear dad. This awesome apple salad is one of our father's favorite snacks, and that is why this recipe is known as Irwin's Waldorf Salad. The apples and raisins lend sweetness to this wonderful salad and the jícama gives it a fresh twist.

1 medium apple, diced (about 1 cup)

2 celery stalks, diced (about 1 cup)

½ cup diced jícama

⅓ cup raisins

⅓ cup chopped walnuts

½ cup plain dairy or nondairy yogurt

¼ cup vegan mayonnaise

1 head Bibb or butter lettuce, washed and leaves separated

Place the apples, celery, jícama, raisins, and walnuts in a large bowl and stir in the yogurt and mayonnaise until well combined. Arrange the lettuce leaves on individual plates or a serving platter, spoon the apple mixture on top, and serve.

IT'S SO GOOD, you're "kidneying" me salad

YIELD: 4 SERVINGS

Kidney beans are a low-calorie, high-protein, fiber-packed food . . . and we're not kidneying!

1 can (15 ounces) kidney beans

5 radishes, sliced thin

½ red cabbage, shredded

1 small yellow bell pepper, seeded and diced

2 small shallots or green onions, chopped fine

2 tablespoons chopped fresh parsley

½ cup pine nuts, toasted

½ cup red wine vinegar

¼ cup extra-virgin olive oil

1 tablespoon Dijon mustard

2 garlic cloves, minced

¼ teaspoon dried oregano

¼ teaspoon sea salt

¼ teaspoon freshly ground black pepper

Place the kidney beans, radishes, red cabbage, bell pepper, shallots, parsley, and pine nuts in a large bowl and stir to mix. Whisk the vinegar, oil, mustard, garlic, oregano, sea salt and black pepper in a separate bowl, then pour over the bean mixture and stir. Place the salad in a large airtight container and refrigerate for at least 2 hours. This mixture is great spooned over butter lettuce leaves.

Homemade Dressings

11

Making your own dressings at home is easy and tasty. We prefer using freshly ground peppers, spices, and herbs, but we cook with dried herbs and seasonings when fresh produce is out of season. Using the freshest ingredients possible will give you the best results.

DRESSINGS

COOL AND CREAMY **italian dressing**

YIELD: 2 CUPS

1 cup extra-virgin olive oil

½ cup red wine vinegar

2 tablespoons fresh lemon juice

2 garlic cloves, minced

1 teaspoon onion powder

1 teaspoon dried basil

1 teaspoon dried oregano

1 teaspoon freshly ground black pepper

½ teaspoon dry mustard

½ teaspoon celery seed

Process all the ingredients in a blender or food processor until smooth. Use immediately or store in the refrigerator for up to 7 days.

lime VINAIGRETTE

YIELD: 1¼ CUPS

You can vary the amount of lime juice in this recipe to suit your taste.

½ cup extra-virgin olive oil

¼ cup red wine vinegar

3 to 4 tablespoons fresh lime juice, from 2 limes

2 tablespoons chopped fresh cilantro

1 garlic clove, minced

¼ teaspoon ground cumin seeds

¼ teaspoon cardamom

¼ teaspoon sea salt (optional)

Place all the ingredients in a medium bowl and whisk to blend, or place in a blender and process until smooth. Use immediately or store in the refrigerator for up to 7 days.

ROQUEFORT **vinaigrette**

YIELD: 1 CUP

3 ounces Roquefort cheese or
nondairy blue cheese substitute

5 tablespoons red wine vinegar

¼ cup extra-virgin olive oil

3 tablespoons dairy or nondairy
sour cream

Process all the ingredients in a blender or food processor until smooth. Use immediately or store in the refrigerator for up to 7 days.

BALSAMIC **vinaigrette**

YIELD: 1½ CUPS

1 cup extra-virgin olive oil

½ cup balsamic vinegar

1 tablespoon chopped fresh parsley

1 garlic clove, minced

½ teaspoon dried basil

½ teaspoon freshly ground black
pepper

Process all the ingredients in a blender or food processor until smooth. Use immediately or store in the refrigerator for up to 7 days.

LEMON **vinaigrette**

YIELD: ¾ CUP

You can vary the amount of lemon juice in this dressing to suit your taste.

½ cup extra-virgin olive oil

3 to 4 tablespoons fresh lemon juice, from 1 to 2 lemons

2 garlic cloves, minced

½ teaspoon paprika

½ teaspoon sea salt (optional)

Process all the ingredients in a blender or place in a medium bowl and whisk until combined. Use immediately or store in the refrigerator for up to 7 days.

HOPE RANCH **dressing**

YIELD: 2 CUPS

1 cup buttermilk

½ cup vegan mayonnaise

½ cup plain dairy or nondairy yogurt

1 tablespoon chopped green onions

2 teaspoons chopped fresh parsley

1 garlic clove, minced

½ teaspoon garlic powder

¼ teaspoon onion powder

¼ teaspoon ground cumin

¼ teaspoon paprika

Process all the ingredients in a blender until smooth. Use immediately or store in the refrigerator for up to 7 days.

yummy lemon TAHINI DRESSING

YIELD: 2 CUPS

¾ cup tahini (roasted sesame seed butter)

⅓ cup fresh lemon juice, from 2 lemons

¼ cup sesame oil

¼ cup tamari

½ medium green bell pepper, chopped

1 celery stalk, chopped

½ yellow onion, chopped

Process all the ingredients in a blender or food processor until smooth. Use immediately or store in the refrigerator for up to 7 days.

VEGAN FRUIT salad dressing

YIELD: 1¾ CUPS

8 ounces firm tofu, mashed

¼ cup canola oil

¼ cup fresh lemon juice, from 2 lemons

¼ cup liquid sweetener of your choice

½ teaspoon vanilla extract

¼ teaspoon ground cinnamon

⅛ teaspoon sea salt, optional

Process all the ingredients in a blender or food processor until smooth. Use immediately or store in the refrigerator for up to 7 days.

POPPY SEED **dressing**

1 cup canola oil

½ cup apple cider vinegar

¼ cup liquid sweetener of your choice

½ green bell pepper, chopped

½ yellow onion, chopped

2 tablespoons prepared mustard

2 tablespoons poppy seeds

1 teaspoon dried thyme

½ teaspoon sea salt, optional

Process all the ingredients in a blender until smooth. Use immediately or store in the refrigerator for up to 7 days.

Papaya Poppy Seed Dressing. Add ¼ cup of diced fresh papaya for a bit of a sweet taste.

Satisfying Soups

12

All these soups can be made ahead and frozen for up to six months.

SOUPS

NANZ'S vegetable stock

YIELD: 6 CUPS

This vegetable stock is named after our beloved Italian grandmother, Giovanna Ziara Muzio, aka "Nanz." It serves as the basis for many of our soups. This recipe can easily be doubled or tripled so you can make large quantities of stock and freeze it.

5 carrots, halved

4 tomatoes, quartered

3 onions, halved

4 celery stalks with leaves, halved

3 sprigs parsley

2 garlic cloves, minced

2 teaspoons sea salt, optional

8 cups water

Place all the ingredients in a large stockpot. Bring to a boil, reduce the heat to low and cover. Let simmer for at least 1 hour. Allow the stock to cool to lukewarm, then strain it through a fine sieve. Discard the vegetables, let the liquid cool to room temperature, then refrigerate or freeze until needed.

BEACHY **barley soup**

Barley is an excellent source of fiber and is known to lower cholesterol.

6 cups Nanz's Vegetable Stock
(page 124), **or other vegetable stock**

¼ cup uncooked, hulled whole
barley, rinsed

1 large carrot, sliced (about 1 cup)

1 cup fresh peas

8 ounces white mushrooms, sliced
(about 1 cup)

1 large onion, chopped (about ¾ cup)

1 celery stalk, diced (about ½ cup)

1 tablespoon tamari

Place the vegetable stock and barley in a large, heavy saucepan, cover, and simmer for 1 hour. Add the carrot, peas, mushrooms, onion, celery, and tamari to the pot, cover, and continue to simmer over low heat for 1 more hour.

Note: Hulled barley is a whole grain with only its outer hull removed; pearled barley has had its bran removed as well, so it is lower in fiber and some nutrients. Pearled barley cooks more quickly, so if you substitute it in this recipe, cook it for just 30 minutes before adding the vegetables.

ENERGIZING **black bean soup**

YIELD: 6 TO 8 SERVINGS

Black beans are rich in antioxidant compounds called anthocyanins, which are also found in fruits such as grapes and cranberries. This fiber-rich food adds a unique texture to soup.

1½ cups dried black beans, picked over and rinsed

3 tablespoons extra-virgin olive oil

1 onion, chopped

2 celery stalks, chopped (about 1 cup)

2 garlic cloves, minced

6 cups Nanz's Vegetable Stock (page 124), or other vegetable stock

1 bay leaf

3 tablespoons nutritional yeast

2 tablespoons whole-wheat flour

1 tablespoon celery seeds

1 tablespoon tamari

½ teaspoon freshly ground black pepper

½ cup fresh lemon juice, from 3 lemons

Heat the oil in a large, heavy-bottomed pot over medium heat, add the onion, celery, and garlic, and sauté for 5 minutes or until the vegetables are slightly softened. Add the vegetable stock, beans, and bay leaf. Bring the mixture to a boil, then cover, reduce the heat, and simmer for 3 hours, or until the beans are tender. Add the nutritional yeast, flour, celery seeds, tamari, and pepper. Purée the soup in batches in a food processor or blender. Return the puréed soup to the pot and reheat, stirring, until the mixture thickens slightly. Stir in the lemon juice and serve.

Note: The bay leaf helps make the beans more digestible.

great GAZPACHO

Gazpacho is served cold, so it's the perfect choice to satisfy a summer craving for soup.

2 cans (16 ounces each) tomato juice

¼ cup red wine vinegar

2 tablespoons fresh lemon juice

2 tomatoes, diced

1 large cucumber, chopped fine

4 green onions, chopped

1 can (6 ounces) sliced black olives, drained

1 avocado, peeled and chopped fine

½ teaspoon garlic powder

½ teaspoon cayenne pepper

2 limes, cut into wedges

Place the tomato juice, vinegar, and lemon juice in a large pot and whisk to blend. Add the tomatoes, cucumber, green onions, olives, avocado, garlic powder, and cayenne and mix well. Cover and refrigerate several hours or overnight. Serve garnished with the lime wedges.

TARYN'S **chilled tomato soup**

YIELD: 5 SERVINGS

This quick and easy soup is so refreshing on a summer day. We like to eat this soup with whole-wheat crackers and low-fat cottage cheese.

3½ pounds ripe tomatoes, peeled and chopped

2 tablespoons extra-virgin olive oil

4 garlic cloves, minced

2 tablespoons balsamic vinegar

½ teaspoon freshly ground black pepper

Place the tomatoes in a blender with the oil and garlic and blend until smooth. Pass the mixture through a sieve to remove the seeds. Stir in the balsamic vinegar and season with the pepper. Refrigerate for 2 hours until chilled, and serve.

CREAMY cauliflower soup

YIELD: 6 SERVINGS

Cauliflower is a cruciferous vegetable like broccoli, kale, and cabbage, all of which have cancer-preventing nutrients. It adds a delicious nutty flavor to this creamy soup.

1 large head cauliflower

5 cups Nanz's Vegetable Stock (page 124), or other vegetable broth

1½ cups cooked pasta bows (farfalle)

14 ounces firm tofu, puréed until smooth

½ cup freshly grated Parmesan cheese or nondairy Parmesan-style cheese

½ teaspoon ground nutmeg

¼ teaspoon sea salt

¼ teaspoon freshly ground black pepper

⅛ teaspoon cayenne pepper

Cut the leaves and central stalk away from the cauliflower and discard. Divide the cauliflower into florets. Bring the vegetable stock to a boil in a large saucepan and add the cauliflower. Simmer for about 10 minutes. Remove the cauliflower with a slotted spoon and process it in a blender. Pour the blended cauliflower back into the stock and add the tofu, ¼ cup of the Parmesan, the nutmeg, salt, pepper and cayenne.

Process the soup in a blender and press through a sieve. Stir in the cooked pasta. Reheat the soup and top each bowl of soup with a little of the remaining Parmesan.

mighty MINESTRONE

YIELD: 10 SERVINGS

This seems to be everyone's favorite soup. Minestrone is loaded with vegetables that are high in vitamin C and fiber.

1 quart water

2 medium carrots, diced small

½ head green cabbage, shredded

1 medium potato, scrubbed and diced

1 can (14.5 ounces) unsalted tomatoes

1 vegetable bouillon cube

2 tablespoons extra-virgin olive oil

1 medium yellow onion, sliced

2 celery stalks, sliced diagonally

1 zucchini, sliced

2 garlic cloves, minced

1 can (15 ounces) navy beans

1 can (8 ounces) tomato sauce

2 tablespoons chopped fresh parsley

½ teaspoon dried basil

½ teaspoon marjoram

½ teaspoon sea salt (optional)

½ teaspoon freshly ground black pepper

Pour the water into a large stockpot. Stir in the carrots, cabbage, potato, tomatoes, and bouillon cube, bring to a boil, then reduce the heat and let simmer. Place the oil in a large skillet over medium heat, add the onion, celery, zucchini, and garlic, and sauté until the vegetables are slightly softened. Add the vegetable mixture to the stockpot. Stir in the beans, tomato sauce, parsley, basil, marjoram, salt (if using), and pepper. Let the mixture simmer over low heat for 30 minutes. Serve hot.

HEARTY BROCCOLI **cheese soup**

Broccoli is a very nutritious vegetable with cancer-preventing properties.

¼ cup water

1 tablespoon fresh lemon juice

2 small bunches broccoli (1½ cups of florets)

1 tablespoon extra-virgin olive oil

1 onion, chopped

2 garlic cloves, minced

3 cups Nanz's Vegetable Stock (page 124), or other vegetable stock

3 large russet potatoes, scrubbed and diced (about 2 cups)

¼ teaspoon ground nutmeg

¼ teaspoon garlic powder

1 cup dairy or nondairy milk

4 ounces Monterey Jack cheese or nondairy Monterey Jack–style cheese, shredded (1 cup)

Pour the water and lemon juice into a small saucepan and bring to a boil over medium heat. Add the broccoli and cook until tender, but still crisp. Drain the broccoli and set aside.

Heat the oil in a large saucepan over medium heat and add the onion and garlic. Sauté until translucent and soft. Add the broccoli, vegetable stock, potatoes, nutmeg, and garlic powder. Bring to a boil, then cover, lower the heat, and simmer for 1 hour. Transfer the soup to a food processor or blender and process in batches until smooth. Return the soup to the pan and add the milk and cheese. Reheat the soup and serve.

CHUMASH **corn soup**

Named for a tribe of Indians who live in our area, this golden soup makes a light but satisfying supper. Try to use the freshest corn because the natural sugars in the kernels quickly begin to convert to starch and the corn becomes increasingly mealy. Even in soup, corn reveals its age and its sweetness!

3 cups Nanz's Vegetable Stock (page 124), **or other vegetable stock**

2 cups fresh corn kernels, from about 6 ears of corn

¼ cup chopped green onions

1 tablespoon tamari

2 garlic cloves, minced

½ teaspoon onion powder

⅛ teaspoon dried mustard

2 cups dairy or nondairy milk

¼ cup shredded Monterey Jack cheese or nondairy Monterey Jack–style cheese

Chopped fresh parsley for garnish

Combine the vegetable stock, corn, green onions, tamari, garlic, onion powder, and mustard in a large saucepan and bring to a boil over medium-high heat. Lower the heat and simmer for 30 minutes. Add the milk and simmer for 5 more minutes. Remove the corn from the soup with a slotted spoon and set aside. Process the soup in a blender or food processor until smooth. Return the soup to the saucepan and add the cheese and corn. Heat the soup for about 10 minutes over low heat, stirring frequently, until the cheese has melted. Serve garnished with chopped parsley.

A Few Basics

Glossary

Agave: Agave nectar is derived from a cactus native to Mexico. It is 90% fruit sugar and slowly absorbed by the body, making this sweetener ideal for people concerned about their blood sugar levels. Agave has a long shelf life and doesn't crystallize like honey. Measure for measure, it is sweeter than sugar, so if a recipe calls for a cup of sugar, use ¾ cup agave.

Flaxseeds: Flaxseeds are high in fiber, lignans and omega-3 fats. Flaxseed meal may be one of the most powerful natural cholesterol controllers yet discovered. Because whole flaxseeds tend to pass through your body undigested, they should be ground in a spice or coffee grinder before using in recipes.

Liquid sweeteners: Recipes that call for liquid sweeteners can be made with maple syrup, agave nectar, or brown rice syrup. Another option that works well in these recipes, although not vegan, is honey.

Margarine: To avoid trans fats, choose nonhydrogenated margarine. We use Earth Balance Buttery Spread, which is vegan. It is sold in 1-pound tubs.

Nondairy cheese: Several types of cheese, including cream cheese, Parmesan cheese, mozzarella, cheddar, and Monterey Jack, come in nondairy form. Some brands of nondairy cheese include casein, a milk protein, so they are unsuitable for vegans; check the ingredient list if you are concerned.

Nondairy milk: Soy milk, rice milk, and almond milk all work equally well in these recipes. Look for organic brands.

Olive oil: We use extra-virgin olive oil, which is cold-pressed, not extracted with chemical solvents like some other oils. Because extra-virgin olive oil is not refined (chemically treated to remove impurities), it's better to buy organic.

Peanut butter (or nut butter): We prefer using dry roasted, creamy, unsalted nut butters in our recipes, except for almond butter, which can be raw or dry roasted. Raw almond butter has a sweet, delicate taste.

Salt: Most of our recipes do not call for salt, or list it as an optional ingredient. We prefer to use herbs to flavor our meals, and many prepared ingredients, such as tomato sauce, mayonnaise, and margarine, already contain salt. If you do add salt when cooking or at the table, we recommend sea salt or kosher salt. Sea salt is obtained by evaporating seawater, and is a pure source of salt (sodium chloride). Kosher salt typically contains no additives, and it gets its name not because it follows the guidelines for kosher foods as written in the Torah, but rather because of its use in making meats kosher. Kosher salt grains are larger than regular salt grains.

Sesame oil: This oil made from sesame seeds is available toasted and untoasted. Untoasted sesame oil has a mild flavor and is suitable for cooking. Toasted sesame oil has a strong, nutty flavor and is best used in small amounts as a flavor accent in salad dressings or drizzled over cooked foods.

Tomato sauce and other canned tomato products: We prefer to use unsweetened, low-sodium tomato sauce. Read labels carefully; often, sauces contain hidden sugars such as high-fructose corn syrup and dextrose. Even organic sauces may contain organic sugar, and there is no need to put sugar in tomato sauce.

Whole-wheat flour: 100% whole-wheat flour is a high-protein flour that includes the bran, germ, and endosperm of the wheat grain. It works well in bread and pizza dough. Whole-wheat pastry flour is made from a softer wheat; its milder flavor and lower gluten content make it more suited to cookies, cakes, and pies.

SEVEN DAY LIGHT-MODERATE-LIGHT MEAL PLAN FOR MAINTAINING YOUR IDEAL WEIGHT

Recently we were at a party and the host came up to us and said, "How do I get legs like you two? " Shari smiled and said, "I guess running, swimming, walking and eating right every day for twenty-five years ought to do it!" The host replied, "Can't I just take a pill that will do it?" We laughed and said, "No!" There are no quick fixes when it comes to your health. It's all about consistency and commitment to a lifestyle. But, as we mentioned before, it is never too late to start eating right and exercising!

Diet pills and weight loss fad diets may have short-term results, but will leave you frustrated when the weight comes back. We don't know the long-term effects of plastic surgery such as liposuction, gastric bypass surgery, or tummy tucks. However, in the short term, any surgery is certainly invasive, expensive and potentially risky.

The Double Energy Diet is a lifestyle. If you want to feel and look good and have more energy, then you have to incorporate this diet into your life. If you follow this regimen, you will achieve your ideal weight. You will develop the ability to choose wholesome foods and you will no longer need to count calories or even worry about portion sizes. We know this is true because we are living proof that this diet works. We always say, "The proof is in the pudding!!" Here's a seven-day plan that incorporates some of the recipes in this book. Here's to you, Beautiful!

Day One

Breakfast: Double Your Energy Health Drink (page 60) with ½ grapefruit

Lunch: Egg-ceptional Eggplant Parmesan (page 91) and a green salad with Balsamic Vinaigrette (page 119)

Dinner: Chumash Corn Soup (page 132) with crackers or croutons

Day Two

Breakfast: Beach Banana Bread (page 70) with fresh strawberries

Lunch: Sunset Sun Burgers (page 99) and a green salad with Roquefort Vinaigrette (page 119)

Dinner: Mighty Minestrone (page 130) and crackers

Day Three

Breakfast: Sunsational Cinnamon Peaches (page 71) with yogurt and toasted almonds

Lunch: Fiesta Combo Pizzas (page 103) with Festival Greek Salad (page 112)

Dinner: California Cool Slaw (page 109) with Hearty Broccoli Cheese Soup (page 131)

Day Four

Breakfast: Wholesome Buttermilk Pancakes (page 75) with fresh fruit

Lunch: Eastside Enchiladas (page 88) with Guacamole Mjelde (page 90)

Dinner: It's So Good, You're "Kidney-ing" Me Salad (page 115) with Delightful Corn Muffins (page 68)

Day Five

Breakfast: Great Granola (page 73) with yogurt or rice milk and fresh fruit

Lunch: Satisfying Stuffed Bell Peppers (page 96)

Dinner: Irwin's Waldorf Salad (page 114) with Great Gazpacho (page 127)

Day Six

Breakfast: Devra's Date Bars (page 74) with yogurt and sliced bananas

Lunch: Tanner's Tasty Tostadas (page 92)

Dinner: Asian Cuke Salad (page 111) with rice cakes

Day Seven

Breakfast: Yummy Apple Flax Muffins (page 63) with Banana Tofu Custard (page 66) and fresh fruit

Lunch: Irresistible Lasagna Roll-Ups (page 95)

Dinner: El Capitan Potato Salad (page 110) and Beachy Barley Soup (page 125)

BUYING CALENDAR FOR FRESH PRODUCE

January: Potatoes, turnips, cabbage, onions, Brussels sprouts, avocados, apples, oranges, tangerines, grapefruit, bananas

February: Potatoes, cabbage, broccoli, celery, Brussels sprouts, apples, oranges, grapefruit, rhubarb

March: Potatoes, broccoli, cabbage, celery, asparagus, avocados, apples, bananas, oranges, grapefruit, rhubarb

April: Potatoes, cabbage, carrots, artichokes, lettuce, asparagus, green peas, avocados, bananas, oranges, grapefruit, pineapple, rhubarb, strawberries

May: Potatoes, onions, lettuce, green beans, green peas, asparagus, various melons, apricots, peaches, cherries, pineapple, strawberries

June: Potatoes, onions, lettuce, green beans, green peas, beets, sweet corn, okra, radishes, tomatoes, apricots, peaches, plums, cherries, nectarines, melons (including watermelon), blueberries, strawberries

July: Cabbage, sweet corn, lettuce, green beans, beets, okra, tomatoes, lemons, peaches, plums, apricots, nectarines, melons, all kinds of berries, grapes

August: Sweet corn, beets, eggplant, okra, lettuce, tomatoes, berries, melons, pears, nectarines, peaches, plums, apricots, grapes

September: Beets, eggplant, okra, artichokes, lettuce, melons, grapes, apples, bananas, peaches, plums, nectarines, pears

October: Cabbage, Brussels sprouts, potatoes, sweet potatoes, turnips, cauliflower, squashes, pumpkins, onions, artichokes, avocados, apples, bananas, pears, grapefruit, oranges, honeydews, grapes, cranberries

November: Potatoes, sweet potatoes, turnips, cauliflower, cabbage, Brussels sprouts, onions, squashes, avocados, apples, pears, bananas, oranges, tangelos, tangerines, grapefruit, grapes, cranberries

December: Potatoes, sweet potatoes, Brussels sprouts, onions, apples, bananas, pears, oranges, tangelos, tangerines, grapefruit, limes, cranberries

Note: Try to buy organic and/or local produce when possible. We suggest only buying domestic produce, too. Some fruits and vegetables aren't grown domestically; if you decide to purchase these products, it's best to buy organic. (For example, most bananas are imported, so we purchase organic bananas.) Produce from other countries may be sprayed with pesticides and may have coats of different types of waxes and preservatives. Always wash your fruits and vegetables!

The Twins' Click Picks

WORTHY WEB SITES

The Internet is an excellent source of information. We've sifted out websites that focus on health, nutrition, and environmental awareness. Many of these worthy web sites have links to other notable sites. Here are a handful we think are worth a click.

www.doubleenergytwins.com This is our website—Judi and Shari Zucker, The Double Energy Twins—which gives helpful tips to maintaining a healthy and energetic lifestyle, and a recipe of the month section that features a nutritious, delicious, easy vegetarian recipe.

www.allrecipes.com This site has a huge collection of recipes, from appetizers to desserts, with special categories for meatless, low-fat, low-sodium and other healthy recipes.

www.cosmeticsdatabase.com This site, called Skin Deep, is a database created by the Environmental Working Group, a nonprofit environmental research group in Washington, D.C. that rates cosmetic products on their safety level. Lower scores are better.

www.decentexposures.com This online clothing company sells organic cotton underwear, exercise wear, and more.

www.greenfusiondesigncenter.com This website features all natural, chemical-free beds and furniture.

www.healthylivingsite.org This site is an excellent source of organic resources. Cathy Silvers, a vegan advocate and former sitcom star, has helpful suggestions on raw vegan foods and cooking classes.

www.naturalhealthmag.com This site promotes its magazine and shares feature articles and current health information.

www.naturalhealthperspective.com This site discusses natural therapies that promote personal health, wellness, and healing through a healthy lifestyle.

www.naturalhealthweb.com A quick and easy guide to natural health and alternative medicine

www.nature.org The site of the Nature Conservancy. This site gives helpful advice on living a green lifestyle. The Nature Conservancy is into protecting nature and preserving life.

www.organicgiftshop.com Organic Gift Shop is a small family-run business that specializes in natural and organic products for babies and children.

www.recipesource.com This site has a vast array of ethnic recipes that experienced chefs check out.

www.sustainabletable.org This site explains what sustainable agriculture is and provides shopping guides to help consumers find sustainably-grown food.

www.veganforum.com This is a message board, with member discussions on all aspects of vegan cuisine, including the basics.

www.vegsource.com Tap into this web site to find answers to everything you are curious about when it comes to being a vegetarian.

www.webhomeopath.com This site contains an interactive feature that lets you type in symptoms and find an appropriate homeopathic remedy.

www.whfoods.org This site promotes a healthier way of eating that's enjoyable and affordable. It lists the nutritional profiles and health benefits of more than a hundred healthful foods.

Bibliography

American Dietetic Association. "Position Paper on the Vegetarian Approach to Eating." Journal of the American Dietetic Association, 77:61 (1980): pp.61-69

Anderson, Bob. *Stretching . . . For Everyday Fitness*. New York: Random House and Shelter Publications, 1980.

Anderson, John J.B., ed. *Nutrition and Vegetarianism: Proceedings of Public Health Nutrition Update May 1981*. Chapel Hill, NC: Health Sciences Consortium, 1982.

Baily, Covert. *Fit or Fat?* Boston: Houghton Mifflin, 1978.

Bielinski, R., Y. Schutz and E. Jéquier. "Energy Metabolism during the Postexercise Recovery in Man." American Journal of Clinical Nutrition. 42 (July 1985): pp. 69-82

Borysenko, Joan. *Minding the Body, Mending the Mind*. Reading, MA: Addison-Wesley, 1987.

Brewster, Letitia, and Michael F. Jacobson. *The Changing American Diet*. Washington, DC: Center for Science in the Public Interest, 1978.

Brody, Jane. *Jane Brody's Nutrition Book*. New York: Bantam Books, 1981. rev. 1987.

Brody, Jane. *Jane Brody's Good Food Book*. New York: W.W. Norton & Co., 1985.

Brody, Jane.*The New York Times Guide to Personal Health*. New York, Avon Books, 1982.

Campbell, Jeremy. *Winston Churchill's Afternoon Nap: A Wide Awake Inquiry into the Human Nature of Time*. New York: Simon & Schuster, 1986:rpt. London: Aurum Press Ltd., 1988.

Charley, Helen. *Food Science*. New York: John Wiley & Sons, 1982.

Chopra, Deepak. *Boundless Energy*. New York: Harmony Books, 1995.

Connor, Sonja L., and William E. Connor. *The New American* Diet. New York: Simon & Schuster, 1986.

Cousins, Norman. *Anatomy of an Illness as Perceived by the Patient*. New York: W.W. Norton & Co., 2005.

DeBakey, Michael, E. et al. *The Living Heart Diet*. New York: Raven Press Books, 1984.

Delgaldo, Nick, Kendell, Shawna. *Grow Young and Slim*. Las Vegas, 2003.

Dane, Elizabeth. *Your Body, Your Diet*. New York: Ballantine Books, 2001.

Dombrowski, Daniel A. *The Philosophy of Vegetarianism*. Amherst: University of Massachusetts Press, 1984.

Dwyer, Johanna, "Wonderful World of Vegetarianism." Nutrition and Vegetarianism: Proceedings of Public Health Nutrition Update May 1, 1981.

Food and Nutrition Board, National Research Council, 1980. Recommended Dietary Allowances, 9th ET. Washington DC: National Academy of Sciences.

Glickman, Rosalene. *Optimal Thinking: How to Be Your Best Self*. New York: John Wiley & Sons, Inc., 2002.

Griffin, H. Winter. *Complete Guide to Vitamins, Minerals and Supplements*. Tucson: Fisher Books, 1988.

Hill, Devra Z. *Rejuvenate: The Scientific Way to Look and Feel Younger Without Drugs or Surgery*. Hollywood, Ca: Irwin Zucker & Daughters, Inc., 1982.

Horton, Edward S. "Introduction: An Overview of the Assessment and Regulation of Energy Balance in Humans." American Journal of Clinical Nutrition, 38 (December 1983): pp.972-77.

Kamen, Betty and Si Kamen. *Kids Are What They Eat*. New York: Arco Publishing, 1983.

Kowalski, Robert E. *The 8-Week Cholesterol Cure: How to Lower Your Cholesterol by Up to 40 Percent Without Drugs or Deprivation*. New York: Harper & Row, 1987.

Lappé, Frances Moore. *Diet for A Small Planet*. New York: Ballantine Books, 1991.

Lissner, Lauren, et al. "Dietary Fat and the Regulation of Energy Intake in Human Subjects." American Journal of Clinical Nutrition, 46 (December 1987): pp. 886-92.

Mann, Jim. "Complex Carbohydrates: Replacement Energy for Fat or Useful in Their Own Right?" American Journal of Clinical Nutrition 45 (May 1983): pp. 453-56.

Mateljan, George. *Healthy Living Cuisine*. Montebello, CA: Health Valley Foods, 1984.

McGee, Harold. *On Food and Cooking: The Science and Lore of the Kitchen*. New York: Scribner, 2004.

Melina, Vesanto, and Brenda Davis. *The New Becoming Vegetarian: The Essential Guide to a Healthy Vegetarian Diet*. Summertown, TN: Healthy Living Publications, 2003.

Miettienen, Tatu A. "Dietary Fiber and Lipids." American Journal of Clinical Nutrition, 45 (May 1987): pp.1237-42

Mindell, Earl. *Earl Mindell's New and Revised Vitamin Bible*. New York: Warner Books, 1979.

Mindell, Earl. *Dr. Earl Mindell's Unsafe at Any Meal: How to Avoid Hidden Toxins in Your Food*. New York: Warner Books, 1987.

Minors, D.S. and J.M. Waterhouse. *Circadian Rhythms and the Human*. Bristol, England: John Wright & Sons, Ltd., 1981.

Murphy, J. "Another Reason for Vegetarianism." Journal of the American Medical Association, 255 (Jan. 3, 1986): pp.666.

Normura, A., L.K. Heilbrun, and G.N. Stemmerman. "Prospective Study of Coffee Consumption and the Risk of Cancer." Journal of the National Cancer Institute, 76 (April 1986): pp.587ff.

Piscatella, Joseph C. *Choices for a Healthy Heart*. New York: Workman Publishing, 1987.

Pollitt, Ernesto, and Peggy Amante, eds. "Energy Intake and Activity." Current Topics in Nutrition and Disease, Volume 11. New York: Alan R. Liss, 1984.

Potter, J.D., and A.J. McMichael. "Diet and Cancer of the Colon and Rectum: A Case Study." Journal of the National Cancer Institute. 76 (April, 1986): pp.557ff.

Robertson, Laurel, Carol Flinders, and Brian Ruppenthal. *The New Laurel's Kitchen*. Berkeley: Ten Speed Press, 1986.

Siegel, Bernie S. *Love, Medicine & Miracles*. New York: Harper & Row, 1986.

Silverstone, Trevor, ed. *Appetite and Food Intake: Report of the Dahlem Workshop on Appetite and Food Intake, Berlin 1975*. Berlin: Abakon Verlagsgesellschaft, 1976.

Smith, Pamela. *The Energy Edge*. Washington, DC: LifeLine Press., 1999.

Spring, B.J. et al. "Effects of Carbohydrates on Mood and Behavior." Nutrition Reviews, 44 (May 1986): 51ff.

Swinney, Bridget. *Eating Expectantly: A Practical and Tasty Approach to Prenatal Nutrition*. Minnetonka, MN: Meadowbrook Press, 2006.

Swinney, Bridget. *Healthy Food for Healthy Kids: An A-to-Z Nutritional Know-How for the Well-Fed Family*. Minnetonka, MN: Meadowbrook Press, 1999.

U.S. Department of Health and Human Services, Public Health Service, National Institutes of Health. Diet, Nutrition & Cancer. Prevention: A Guide to Food Choices. NIH Publication No. 85-2711, November 1984.

Zi, Nancy. *The Art of Breathing*. New York: Bantam Books, 1986.

Zucker, Judi and Shari Zucker. *Double Your Energy With Half the Effort*. Norfolk, VA: Hampton Roads Publishing, 1991.

Index

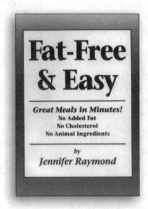
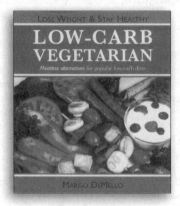
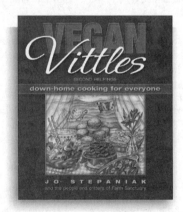
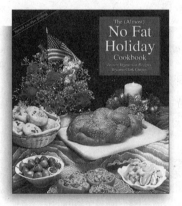